Table of Contents

Debbie Portell
- What made you a Trainer....3
- What are your strengths....5
- Weaknesses....6
- Nutrition Philosophy....6
- Favorite Recipes....10
- Supplements....15
- Workout Schedule....16
- Passion, Heart, Success....17
- Motivation....18
- Train to Live meaning....19
- Style of Training....20
- Favorite Quotes....22
- Client Testimony....24

Bill Clark
- Road to Recovery....32
- The Journey....33
- Nutrition Philosophy....34

John Morris
- What made you a Trainer....35
- What are your strengths....35
- Weaknesses....35
- Nutrition Philosophy....36
- Supplements....36
- Workout Schedule....37
- Passion, Heart, Success....37
- Motivation....38
- Style of Training....39
- Why Choose Integrity....40
- Client Testimony....41

Lisa Klaus-Ogden
- What made you a Trainer....42
- What are your strengths....43
- Weaknesses....43
- Nutrition Philosophy....44
- Supplements....44
- Workout Schedule....44
- Train to Live meaning....45
- Style of Training....46
- Favorite Recipes....47
- Client Testimony....48

Mike Harris
- What made you a Trainer....50
- What are your strengths....50
- Weaknesses....51
- Nutrition Philosophy....51
- Supplements....52
- Workout Schedule....52
- Passion, Heart, Success....53
- Motivation....53
- Train to Live meaning....53
- Client Testimony....54

Misti Weatherford
- What made you a Trainer....59
- What are your strengths....61
- Weaknesses....61
- Nutrition Philosophy....
- Supplements....
- Workout Schedule....
- Passion, Heart, Success....
- Motivation....66
- Style of Training....67
- Favorite Quotes....70
- Why Choose Integrity....71
- Client Testimony....72

Forrest Boston
- What made you a Trainer....74
- What are your strengths....75
- Nutrition Philosophy....76
- Favorite Recipes....78
- Supplements....78
- Workout Schedule....79
- Passion, Heart, Success....81
- Train to Live meaning....82
- Style of Training....84
- Favorite Quotes....92
- Client Testimony....93

Mike Stout
- What made you a Trainer....96
- What are your strengths....96
- Nutrition Philosophy....97
- Supplements....97
- Workout Schedule....98
- Passion, Heart, Success....98
- Train to Live meaning....99
- Style of Training....99
- Favorite Quotes....102
- Client Testimony....103

Mike Lumia
- What made you a Trainer....105
- What are your strengths....106
- Nutrition Philosophy....107
- Favorite Recipes....107
- Supplements....108
- Workout Schedule....108
- Passion, Heart, Success....108
- Motivation....109
- Train to Live meaning....109
- Style of Training....110
- Favorite Quotes....111

Casey Owens
- What made you a Trainer....112
- What are your strengths....113
- Nutrition Philosophy....114
- Favorite Recipes....115
- Supplements....115
- Workout Schedule....116
- Passion, Heart, Success....116
- Motivation....117
- Train to Live meaning....118
- Style of Training....118
- Favorite Quotes....119

"A legacy isn't only about leaving what you have earned but also what you've learned"
-Author unknown

What made you a trainer?
Debbie Portell

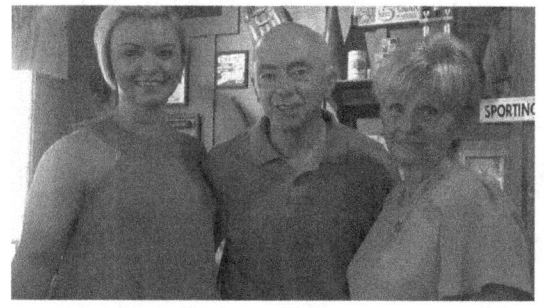

I decided to become a trainer almost 15 years ago. My health declined significantly. After visiting 22 different doctors we determined I have Hashimoto's disease. An auto immune disease of the thyroid. I spent years seeking a diagnosis and suffered everyday along the way. Weight loss and weight gain along with extreme symptoms that were debilitating.

I finally found a team of doctors that was willing to work with me and truly made a difference. The biggest difference came from changing my food. That was the integral part of my life change. I completely eliminated dairy, gluten, soy, corn, pork, shellfish, peanuts and sugar. I was a completely different person from it.

I have worked out since I was a young child. Ever since I can remember I wanted to be just like my dad. He was always working out. He rode bikes, played team sports, ran, played hockey and lifted weights. I always wanted to do whatever he was doing and I did. I even learned to play hockey. On ice! We started lifting weights in the 6th grade. I've been taught by him and some of the best trainers in town. In 8th, 9th and 10th grade I was blessed to have the opportunity to workout at George Turners Gym. I haven't been in a gym like that ever since. Powerhouse played a close second but George Turner and his iron factory was one of a kind. The gym probably had less than 10 females in it much less teenage women. His squat cage had a 45lb plate that remained in it. I guess if you cannot squat that you don't have any business squatting he thought. I was so fortunate to learn from such hard working amazing people.

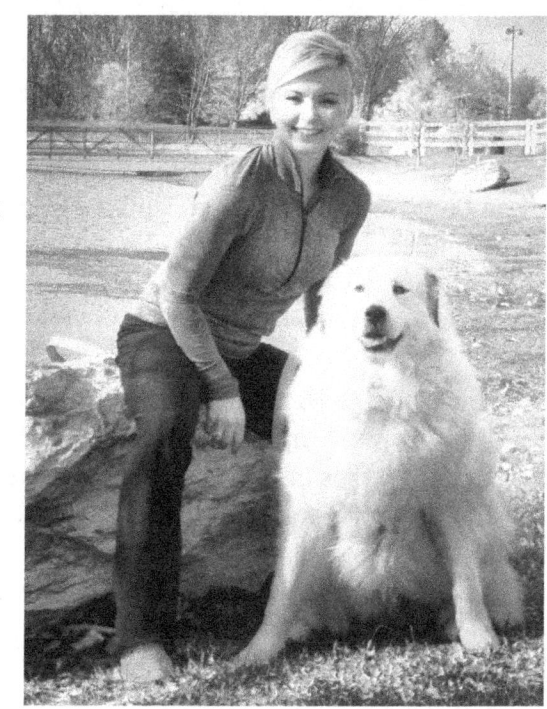

Body building was different back then. It was real. It was not about who you know and how many drugs you can buy. It was about how hard you worked. They ate real food and a lot of it but clean food. They were not constantly popping pills and powders. Only what was important like vitamins and minerals. If you are not sure what I mean just look up a picture of George Turner. We hang his picture in our gym. His physique looks chiseled like a sculpture. He doesn't look like some over inflated giant super hero. The sport had really taken a unique turn.

After George closed his gym we moved to Powerhouse. It was a great gym as well. It started to become a little bit more about leotards and the sexiness of the sport than it was at Turners. Heck I remember the strongest guy at Turners gym wore jean shorts or cargo pants with a flannel shirt no sleeves and boots. Ever since then each gym I moved to became a little bit more about how you look and how quick you could do it versus how hard you were willing to work.

I spent 12 years with Powerhouse gym and Roger Semsch. He is one of the hardest working people in the industry. He has always prepped people to have a healthy life not to just look good. He has always taught me that I get what I give. If I work hard day in and day out I will reap a benefit. If I give 50% I will get 50%. I have truly had the opportunity to learn from amazing people and they have helped me to become who I am today. The first one was my Dad though. He was my first motivator. The first person I could follow. My Mom supported us both through it all. She worked 2 jobs to help me afford my hobbies. She was always there to cook for us and cheer us both on. She still is. Dad and I are very lucky to have her.

When I decided to become a trainer I knew I could really motivate people to live differently. I wanted to inspire them to change their spirit. The focus they put on how they cared for the body and the way they viewed it had to change. I have worked as a trainer in all possible capacities but no matter what the environment I've always been so driven to keep people from settling for status quo. I found that no matter what location I was working out of at least half of the trainers hated me. Ha ha. No really they did. At 5 am when they were leaning and drinking coffee while training looking like they came to work in pajamas I was perky and excited to help my client. I also always had make up on and tried to look presentable. Over time other clients would watch me and my clients train. Enthusiasm is contagious. You can sincerely download it into people. You can also download defeat and garbage into someone.

I have worked at Renaud Spirit Center, General Motors Fitness Center, 24 Hour Fitness, Powerhouse Gym, Rhino Fitness, Complete Fitness, Ladue Pt, Anytime Fitness and all of those places birthed Integrity. I've worked at 4 gyms at one time before. They were all over town. I remember for 3 years making an hour drive to and from to train a client I trained for 8 years just because she was such a hard worker. I drove through sleet, rain and snow to get to her and to all of my clients. I've worked sick and I've worked very tired. I just do my best to hide behind my smile and keep my clients going where they need to go.

I feel I am an old school, body building, strength training trainer that was baptized in functional movement and mobility. I combined all of it together and that is how we train at Integrity. I learned half way through my athletic sports career that if I don't focus on flexibility I will never achieve 100% of what I was seeking. Rather that was speed, strength or agility the foundation of it all was flexibility and mobility. I train every trainer and every client to be this way. Another thing I do different than most is I keep everyone in the best shape they can be in. We jump rope on shoulder day. We use the rowing machine on back day. We flip tires on arm day. We sprint and run stairs on leg day. There is no excuse for not staying cardiovascularly fit. It will benefit you in everything you do if you start. Just start moving anyway that you can. Slow movement is better than no movement.

I sincerely love what I do and I live for it. I live for the Lord first but the beautiful thing is that I am walking in his presence everyday on the job. He directs my words and my actions everyday. I try so hard to stay faithful to him in all that I do and all that we do at Integrity. I jump out of bed to do what I do because I work with amazing people. They never give up on me. They always give me all they have. I always have a group of people that have give up on life and themselves and I jump out of bed begging God for his will to be done but praying that very day would be the day for their turn around. The day they end their love affair with food. The day they look in the mirror and like what they see or the most important the day they surrender their hearts and life to the Lord. Without Jesus we will never be satisfied. We will wonder lost forever. This gym is more than a gym. It is a ministry and each person is there for a season. A life changing, spirit strengthening season ordained by God. I am blessed to be part of it.

What are your strengths?

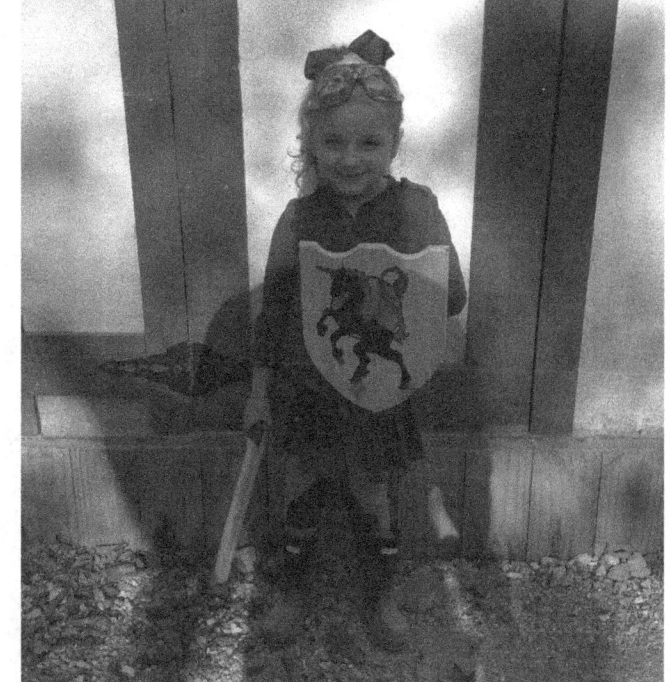

I would say my strength is my Faith and my will to never give up. 15 years ago when I felt I was on my death bed I sincerely refused to die. I saw our Pastor Jeff Perry on the TV talking about hope and asking people to surrender their life to God. I thought well that is the only thing I have not done. I gave my heart to the Lord that very day. I agreed to put him first in all things. I read the Bible from beginning to end. I did this multiple times. I started to attend church. Sometimes I was carried into the church because I was so weak. Other times I couldn't even stand when everyone else was standing.

I just sat and cried and begged God for the strength to stand. Now look at how strong I am! He answers prayer! I believe that my Faith in God is my strongest attribute. I have been manipulated, mistreated, disrespected, stomped on and drug through the mud by many people in my life. Never by the Lord. He has never left me. He has never given up on me. He has always heard my cry. I am never alone. He is always by my side. I would be positively lost and worthless if it wasn't for my faith in Christ.

Weaknesses?

From a weakness stand point I feel I don't have a great deal of compassion for laziness. I feel everyone has the opportunity to change and to redeem them self but I truly feel laziness is a sign of weakness. I believe it contradicts all that God has asked of us in his word. I don't have much compassion for someone who puts off what they could do today for tomorrow. I don't respect someone who makes excuses for why they can't get where they want to go. I don't nurture and baby someone who wants to take the easy way out in life. I wish I could have more compassion. I really do. I just wasn't raised this way. I've spent my entire life surrounded by amazing examples of work ethic. It is all that I know. Unfortunately not everyone else has. Some folks need to be led. They need to be taught as well. They need to be shown what it takes to work hard, to be efficient and to remain driven. I pray daily that God will make me more compassionate and willing to lead and not judge.

My goal is sincerely to live the healthiest life possible. I pray my life is truly a living testimony to that which God wants me to represent. I pray that I can stay strong no matter what temptation I am faced with. I truly hope that my life will cause someone to want to make a decision to be healthier. I pray that I can help people see how deadly food can be as well as how healing it can be.

What is your philosophy on nutrition?

My philosophy on nutrition is that you should eat real, whole food. If you cannot understand the words in the ingredients on what b you are eating neither will your body. You sincerely will find yourself with a disease faster than you know it. Trust me, I know first hand. I ate fake food, processed food and garbage for years. Growing up mom and Dad had a garden. My Grandfather was president of the stock yards. We had meat all the time and fresh vegetables. We didn't eat fake processed packaged foods. As soon as I was out of the house which was at 18 I started eating horrible. Hot dogs, sugared oat meal and cereal, processed bars, fake meats, sugar, sugar and more sugar. Then my body just shut down. Completely!

The statement you are what you eat truly couldn't be more truth to me. I watch people daily fight with symptoms they wouldn't even deal with if they just ate clean. If they avoided gluten, sugar, dairy, corn or processed foods. We have no problem taking a medicine with awful chemicals but we fight tooth and nail against removing poisonous foods from out life. Food is the fuel that will guide and direct your brain, your strength, your attitude and your desire for life. Make your choices wisely.

I do an intermittent fasting diet. You can read more about that on Dr Mercola's website by visiting www.mercola.com and researching intermittent fasting. It has truly changed my life. Roger lost 100 lbs in less than a year by just this one principal. I start eating at 11 and end at around 8. I do my cardio fasted in the morning and I feel great. An example of my day is:

12:00 pm
Meal 1
3 oz grass fed beef
1/4 cup mushrooms
1/2 cup rice cauliflower
1 cup roasted zucchini
1 tbsp Mct Oil

3:00 pm
Meal 2
1 cup of coffee or fresh cucumber juice
1/2 tbsp coconut oil
2 scoops of Collagen protein
1 cup cucumber
1 tbsp Avocado

7:00 pm
Meal 3

Meal Planning

3 oz Boneless Skinless Turkey Breast
1/2 cup rice cauliflower
1 cup green beans roasted
1/2 tbsp Mct oil

9:00 cup of decaf tea with 1/2 tbsp mct oil or 1 cup of beef bone broth.

This is truly how I eat on a very regular basis. As a treat I do about half cup pumpkin seeds on my days off. I don't do fruit or high starch veggies. I would highly recommend reading the book Keto-Adapted for more information on how to eat low carb successfully and why, or call me! I can help.

Sugar is a fuel I do not wish for my engine to run off. When I switched from using sugar for energy to fat for energy I lost 15 lbs and had not lost weight in easily 6 years. My body was so inflamed. Luckily with the help of Dr. Mary Krueter at Bone Chiropractic I was able to determine what foods were not being received well by my body. At least at this time. That will always be ever changing. Right now I avoid eggs, chicken and nuts. I will not forever. There will be a day they won't cause me as much harm but for now I avoid them and feel great because of it.

I eat out every weekend. I just order what I can have. Hamburger or steak with all the veggies they can fit on a plate. Most of the time I bring my own Mct oil to add to it as well as a tea bag and stevia for afterwards. Never underestimate the power of a cup of coffee or tea after a meal with a small amount of coconut oil to curb your appetite and help to make you feel sustained and satisfied.

I see Dr. Mary every other week. She keeps my immune system strong. I see Dr. Ian McDonald every 6 weeks. He does a wonderful job of keeping my structure in check. I see Dr. Richard Bligh every 4 months. He helps me to keep my thyroid and hormone levels in check.

People often ask me what do you feed Sophie. Parents struggle enough to change their own food but then to change a child's food on top of it can be very difficult. I truly believe over time kids will want to do what you do so the best way to change your kids food is to live it out in front of them. They will adapt. Sophie does not complain about her food and she knows what she eats is good for her. She also knows what is not good for her. We have treats along the way but we don't over do it. If we eat cookies they are gluten free. If we have a bar it is gluten free. If we do pizza it is gluten free. If we do ice cream it is coconut milk or almond milk. The inflammation in her gut as well as her allergies have decreased significantly because of these changes. If Sophie has gluten, sugar, corn or dairy. She swells. Even her face swells. Her belly is hard and she has a difficult time going potty. Food matters folks. Not just for adults. It matters for your children too. We always avoid juice, soda, candy, milk, bread and corn. This has helped a great deal. Sophie has also visited with Dr. Mary and we identified that she has a sensitivity to gluten, dairy and sugar. I think everyone does really. A day in the life of Sophie Morris looks like:

Meal 1
1 to 2 scrambled eggs
1 cup strawberries and blueberries

Meal 2
6 dried apricots
15 cashews

Meal 3
2 to 3 oz Lean Turkey
Celery Sticks
8 olives
1 Mandarin orange

Meal 4
Gluten Free Brown Rice Bar or Fruit Based Lara bar

Meal 5
2 to 3 oz Ground Turkey or Ground Beef
unsweetened ketchup
1 cup baked green beans with olive oil

Meal 6
celery and peanut butter, cashew butter or almond butter

Sophie drinks water, hint water, and coconut or almond milk.

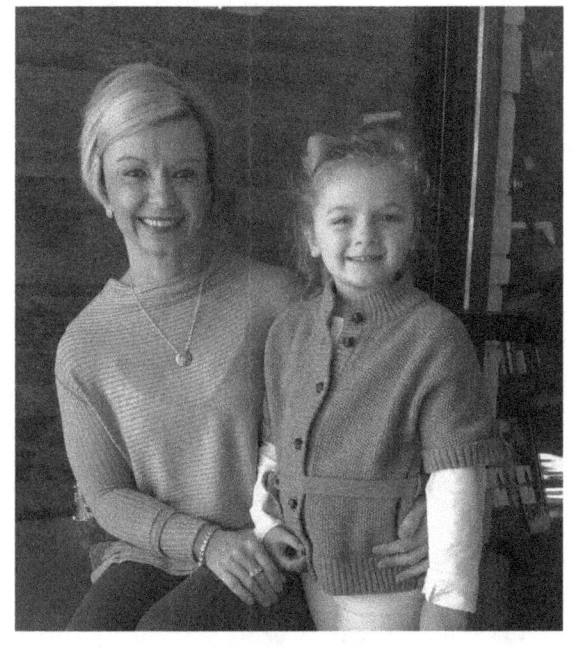

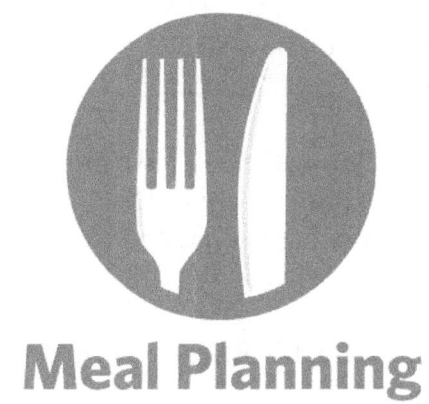

My favorite recipes:

Protein Latte: Makes 12 oz of coffee
1/2 tbsp coconut oil
1/2 tsp raw cacao powder
2 scoops Collagen Protein Powder
2 tbsp unsweetened Coconut Milk
Stevia to taste.

Blend until well blended and enjoy a great way to start the day!

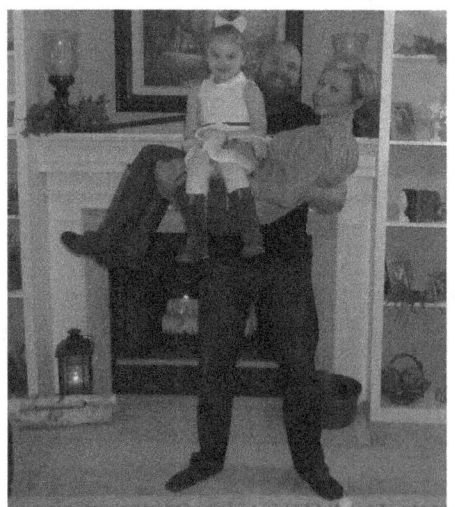

Brussels Sprouts:
2 - 3 lbs. of fresh brussels sprouts (cut in half)
1 large shallot
1 tbsp olive oil
sea salt
pepper
1 tbsp of onion powder
2 cloves of garlic, minced

Saute shallot, garlic and olive oil. Roll fresh Brussels Sprouts in the mixture. Foil line a sheet cake pan, lay veggie mixture out evenly. Bake at 350 for 30
minutes, toss them around and cook 15 minutes more, or until desired doneness.

Grandma Barb's Baked Green Beans:
5 steam in a bag green beans
4 tbsp extra virgin olive oil
1 tbsp pepper
Cook all bags together in microwave for 25 minutes. Spread across foil lined sheet cake pan. Hand kneed the
olive oil so that all beans are covered sprinkle pepper over the top. Cook for 40 minutes on 350. Turn oven off and let rest in oven for 5 to 10 minutes or until desired.

Daily juice
1 cucumber
1 handful parsley
4 stalks celery
1/2 lemon
1/2 tbsp mct oil or chia seeds

Meat Loaf:
3 lbs grass fed beef
3 cups Unsweetened ketchup
1 cup riced cauliflower
1/3 cup spicy guacamole
2 cups chopped mushroom sautéed
2 cups chopped white onion sautéed

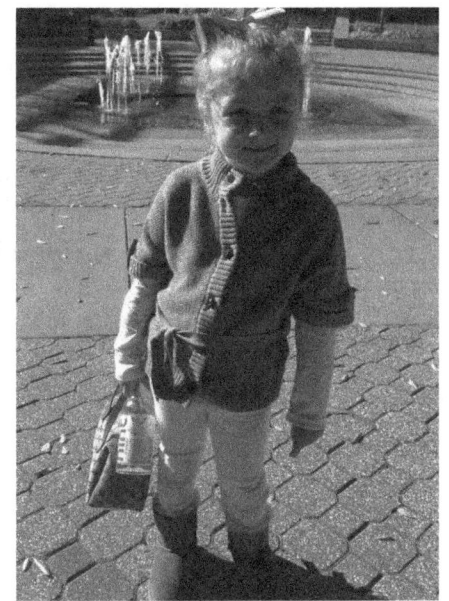

Combine every thing in a large bowl with half the ketchup. Make individual loaves out of the meat mixture. Top with ketchup. Place a cooling rack inside a baking sheet. Set each loaf on top of the cooling rack and top with remaining ketchup. Cook for 1 hour on 325 degrees. Turn oven off. Let remain in oven for 15 minutes longer. It's better the second day!

Crock Pot Green Beans
6 bags frozen green beans
6 tbsp olive oil
6 tsp sea salt
3 tsp pepper

Take green beans one bag at a time and place in a large crock pot with 1 tbsp olive oil, 1 tsp sea salt and 1/2 tsp pepper. Repeat each bag until complete. Cool on low for 6 to 8 hours or until desired doneness.

Cinnamon Apple Yogurt
4 Fuji or honey crisp apples
1 tbsp coconut oil or 2 tbsp olive oil
1 tbsp cinnamon
1 tsp alcohol free vanilla
1 cup unsweetened coconut milk yogurt
1 tsp pure stevia

Chop all apples or use an apple peeler. Leave skin on. Saute them with all ingredients for about 15 minutes or until desired doneness. Serve as dessert with 1 cup unsweetened coconut milk yogurt. You can add more cinnamon and stevia as needed.

Dairy Free Yogurt Protein Smoothie:
1 scoop strawberry protein
1 cup mixed berries thawed with juice
1 tbsp flavored flax oil
1/2 tsp pure stevia
1/2 tbsp chia seeds

Blend all ingredients and serve. All ingredients can be added to an ice cream maker with more unsweetened coconut milk and you have healthy protein packed ice cream!

Deviled eggs:
12 hard boiled eggs
2 Avocado cubed
1 tbsp mct oil
2 tbsp chopped chives
1 tsp sea salt
1/2 tsp pepper
1 pinch of cayenne
1 tsp yellow mustard
1/2 tbsp apple cider vinegar

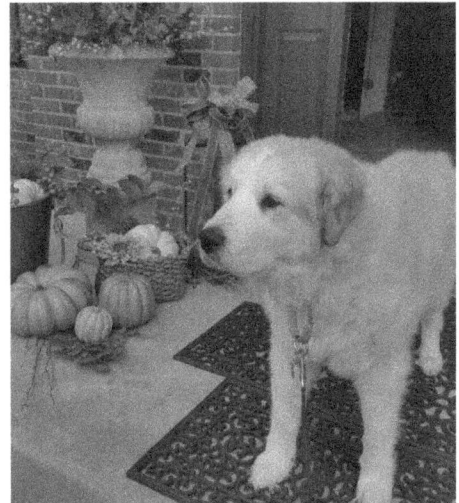

Blend all ingredients along with egg yolk. Add to a large ziploc bag. Cut a snip of the end of the bag and pipe the egg mixture into the hard boiled egg whites.

Pumpkin Spice Protein Latte
1 tbsp pumpkin spice coconut butter
1 tsp coconut butter
Dash of pure stevia
Dash of Cinnamon
Dash of alcohol free vanilla
2 scoops Collagen protein.
Blend all ingredients with 10 to 12 oz of coffee and enjoy!

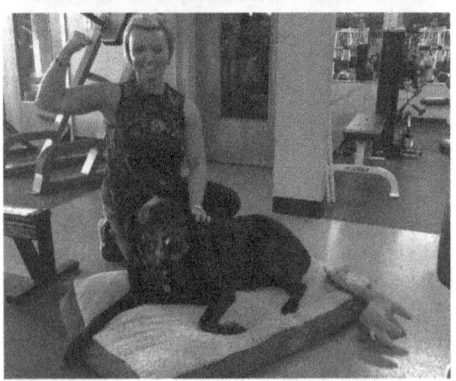

Green Tea Latte
10 oz of green tea hot steeped
1/2 tbsp lemon coconut butter
1/2 tbsp coconut oil
Dash of stevia
Dash of cinnamon
2 scoops of Collagen protein

Blend all ingredients together and enjoy!

Pan Fried Green Beans:
1 steam in the bag great beans
2 tbsp olive oil
1 small chopped shallot
Sea Salt and pepper to taste

Microwave the green beans for 6 minutes. Saute shallot in 1 tbsp olive oil. When cooked add the steamed green beans and additional olive oil. Stir constantly and cool on medium until the start to brown on at least one side. They are my French fries!

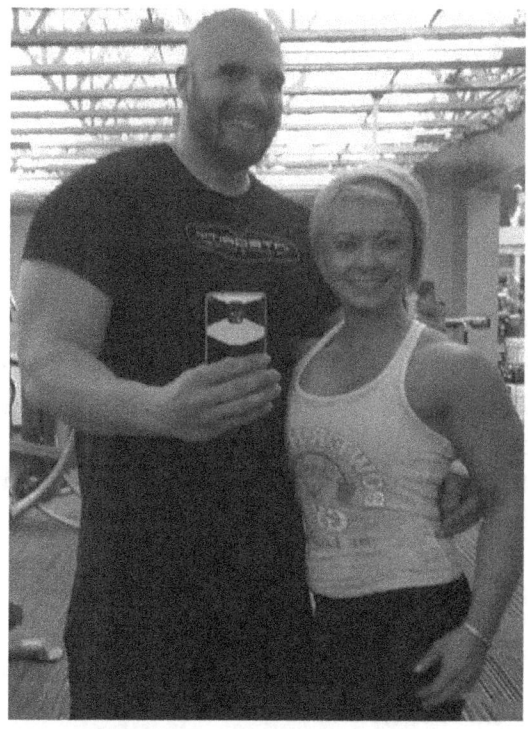

Cinnamon Cashew Butter:
1 large tub of Pure Plates cashew butter
1 tbsp cinnamon
1/2 tsp sea salt
1 tsp alcohol free vanilla
1 tbsp coconut oil

Add all ingredients to your blender until combined. Great on celery or Sophie will eat it with an apple. Also good on top of my cinnamon vanilla egg white pancake.

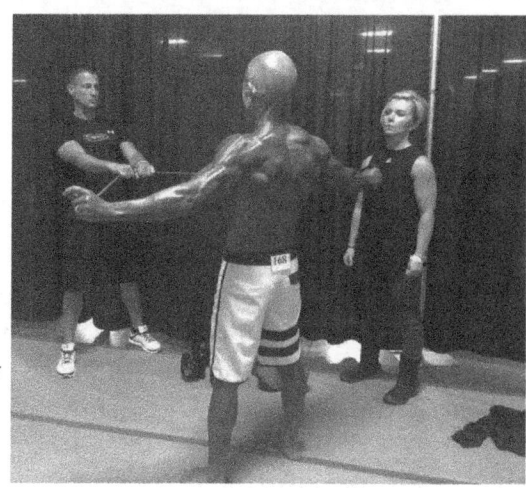

Crunchy Dijon Salmon:
2 lbs of Pure Plates Salmon
1 tsp sea salt
1/2 tsp pepper
1 tbsp minced onion
1 cup mustard vinaigrette Simple Girl Dressing
1 tbsp olive oil

Combine all ingredients except olive oil and pour on top of salmon. Heat your olive oil on medium in a skillet. Cast iron works best. Heat up the pan first. You want to hear a sizzle when you add the salmon. Add the already cooked Pure Plates salmon mixture to the heated skilled. Pan fry the salmon until it has a desired crust. I serve it with baked green beans.

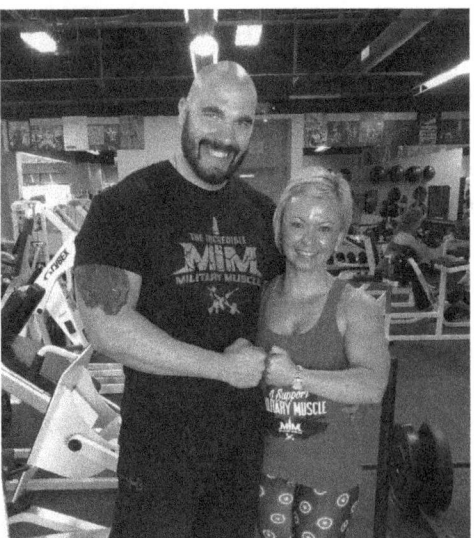

Coconut Chocolate Bar Fat Bombs:
1 cup unsweetened, shredded coconut
1 packet of stevia
1 tsp vanilla extract
1/2 cup coconut cream
4 tbsp coconut oil
2 tbsp unsweetened cocoa powder
OPTION-instead of coconut oil for the coating 2 oz cocoa butter

Mix shredded coconut with coconut cream, 1/2 of the vanilla extract and 1/2 packet of stevia and blend well with a spatula or a spoon. Place the shredded coconut mixture on a small cookie sheet lined with parchment paper. Shape it into a flat rectangle about 4 inches by 6 inches and 1 inch thick (measurements may vary). You can aid yourself with kitchen wrap to accomplish this. Place in the freezer for 2 hours until frozen solid. Remove from the freezer and cut into 5 bars. In the meantime you will prepare the chocolate coating. Melt coconut oil in a small sauce pan until liquefied. Add cocoa powder remaining stevia and vanilla

Sweet and spicy mustard
1/2 cup yellow mustard
1 tbsp Franks hot sauce
2 dash pure stevia

Combine all ingredients. I dip everything into it.

Do you take supplements?

I take supplements daily. Both Dr Mary and Dr Bligh have been instrumental in helping to know what works best. Most of my supplements are for immune system support, electrolyte balance, building energy in the mitochondria, improving gut bacteria and balancing estrogen. I take all of my pills and separate them on Sunday night. I put them in small baggies and bring them with me. Since I fast I wait until 11 until I start taking them. I take 3 or 4 at a time each time I eat. I do take 90mg of Armor Thyroid. I take this as soon as I wake up with water. My daily supplements include:

Lcarnitine
Estrofactors
Xvironmin
ALA
Probiotic
Vitamin d
Magnesium
Potassium
Endurolytes
Vitamin

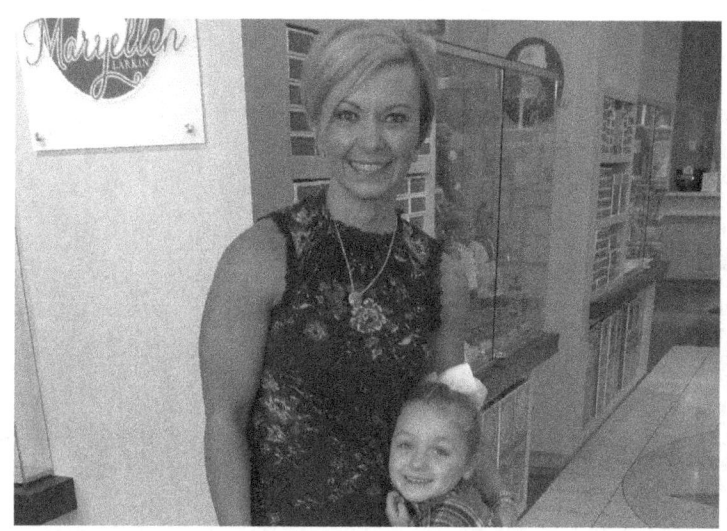
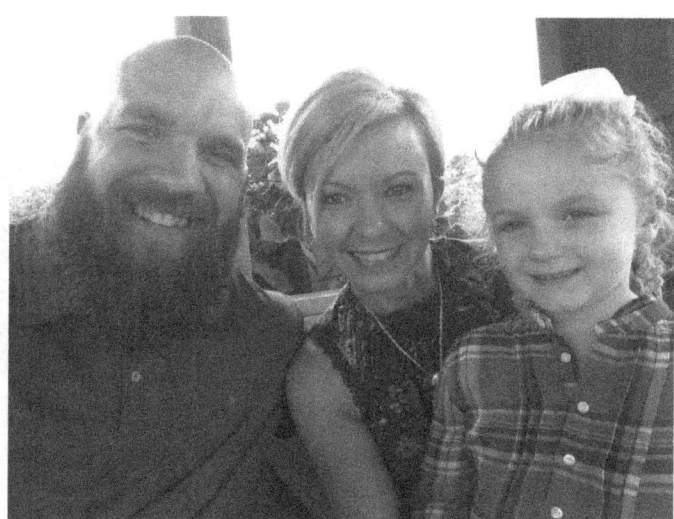

What is your workout schedule & why?

My workout schedule is pretty consistent but has changed a bit recently after losing the weight and dropping so much inflammation. My body has never had a problem putting on muscle. However it's always had a problem dropping body fat. My lifts have changed recently. I'm doing more of a full body focus and I am concentrating on getting extra cardio in. My work week looks like this:

Wednesday 12 to 13 hours
Thursday 10 hours
Friday 12 hours
Saturday 9 hours
Sunday 8 hours
Monday and Tuesday off days. I work on paperwork at home.

I wake up each day and start with cardio. 30 minutes on my octane elliptical at home. I do this everyday but Saturday fasted in the am. I lift Sunday after work and do an additional 30 minutes of cardio after the lift. I also lift on Monday and Tuesday and do an additional 30 minutes of cardio on those days as well. I have 1 rest cardio day. 3 lift days and 3 days of the week that I do cardio twice.

My lifts are Sunday bicep and triceps. Monday back and shoulders and Tuesday legs. Over the years I have done every type of workout imaginable. There is no one workout that is best for anyone. I think life changes. I think our health changes. I think we have to be ready to adapt as that changes. Over working yourself when you are already broken down will only make the situation worse. I've learned that the hard way. The

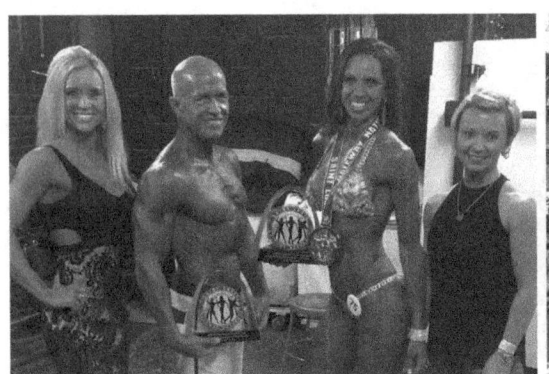
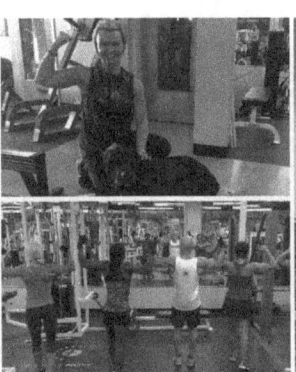
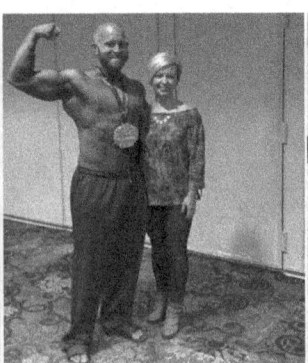
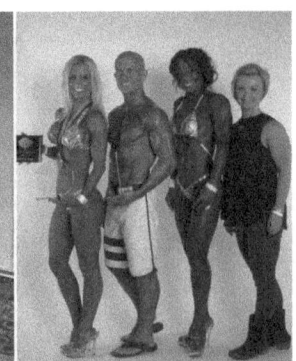

body needs rest. You must sleep. Without it you will remain swollen. Your lymph system will not drain properly. This means that toxins will stay stuck in your body. That doesn't help anyone. That is what over training means. I've also had seasons where I trained 2 to 3 hours a day 6 days a week. I slept every night. I restored. I stretched and foam rolled. I had a massage every 4 weeks and I saw Dr Ian my chiropractor regularly. Over training comes not because you workout too much but because you are missing the other key components. You must sleep, eat, hydrate and work on your flexibility. All of these need to be scheduled.

What is your definition of passion? Heart? Success?

I truly believe passion is not something you are born with. I feel it is bread in you. My parents taught me it. They showed me through years of hard work. Passion is the fuel that keeps you ignited until you finally accomplish what you have set out to achieve. Without passion life is flat. However until you find your purpose and you decide to walk with purpose you will never find your passion.

Eric Thomas always talks about heart. He says you can get up and do the work like everyone else. However someone with HEART will always out work you. The heart for the game for life or for success it what catapults a person ahead of others. When you see people that are on different level. Maybe it's a level you aspire to be at. The main thing you can see different about them is first they have heart. That goal or that drive is embedded in them. They refuse to give up and it's their passion that keeps the heart driving forward no matter how hard it gets.

Success is not about a title, money, houses or cars. I've had it all and felt lonely and lost. Success is about peace. It's about joy. It's about living in the sweet spot. Even during the tough times you refuse to not give up. You count it all joy and you continue to serve God and you give him the glory when you achieve. Success is truly when you find a way to look in the mirror and say I am enough. I will work to be better and I will serve God but I am enough. You stop caring about social media. You stop caring about what the critics say. You stop caring about what the bank account says. You serve God day in and day out and he is your provider. He is your bank account. His opinion is what matters. Your focus and your time is on increasing him. Success comes when you realize it's not about you it's about HIM.

How do you stay motivated to make this a lifestyle and not a goal?

My strongest motivation to make this a lifestyle is my health. If I don't stay committed to my food I will be sick. I can be sick within 30 minutes of eating something. I've spent time in the emergency room just because of one wrong food. One wrong seasoning. One wrong oil. I don't have a choice but to make this a lifestyle. I tried many years ago to eat anything I wanted whenever I wanted and I almost died.

Most people don't realize how much the food they eat is effecting how they feel daily. Being told you have type 2 diabetes, high blood pressure or is a rough thing to hear. What if the doctor told you that you could cure all of that with your food? What makes 50% of the population choose not to change even though they know the food they are eating is causing the disease. Is it because they are addicted? Is food their drug? Possibly. It can change. Meet with someone that can teach you how to adapt and change your food. You can live disease free. You can be freed of food addiction. You are the one making the choices. Choose to work towards progress not perfection. Stop putting poison in your body and in your children. Start standing on the principle that your body is a temple of the Holy Spirit that God had given you. Bless that temple. It is the only one you will ever be given.

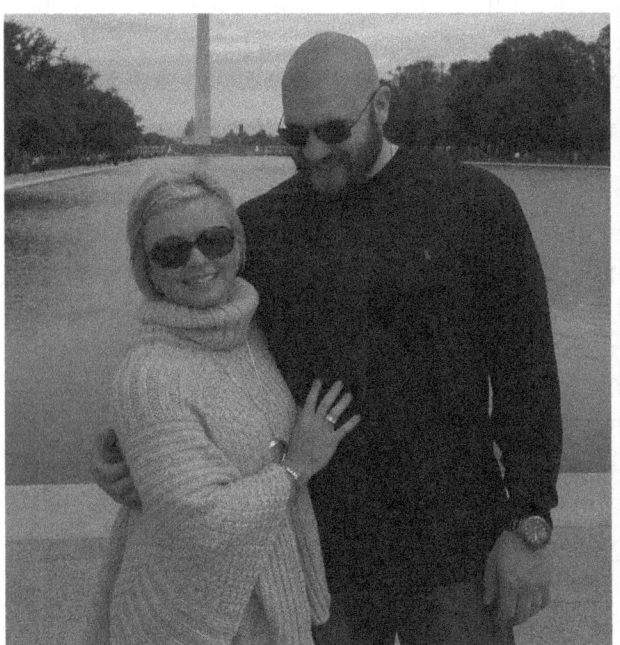
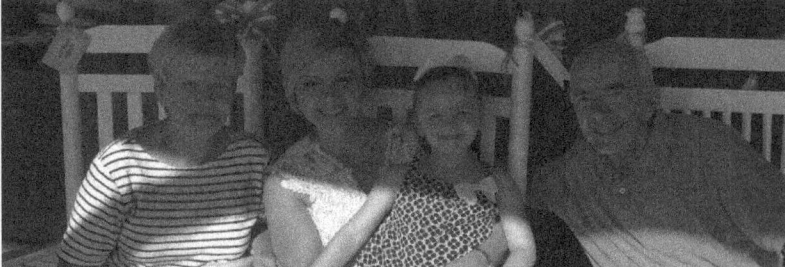
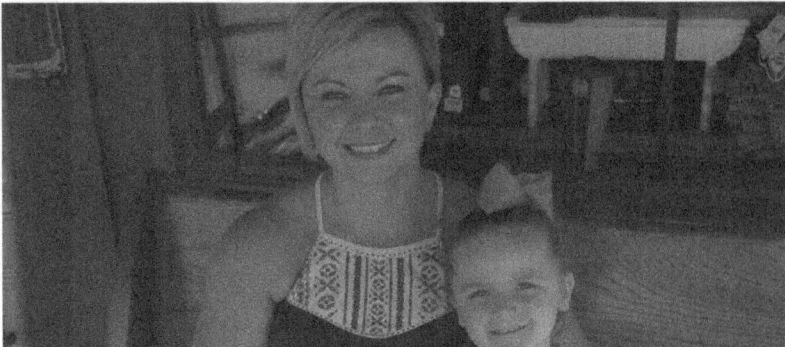

What does Train to Live mean to you?

Train to Live means know your WHY. Why do you train? What is your purpose? Train to Live a healthy lifestyle. Train to be better at your job, better for your family and most importantly to feel your very best. Training to look good is great. I respect it but it'd hollow. It won't last. You will make sacrifices. You will take fat burners, drink energy drinks, eat the wrong foods if it helps you to look better. You won't sustain those results and you won't be healthy. LIVE is the ultimate word. Food is life or death for you. Activity done properly and consistently can help keep you well forever. If your desire is to be faster, stronger and leaner than stop making excuses. Stop taking short cuts. As Eric Thomas says don't go to sleep until you succeed. Lastly Emmitt Smith one of my favorite players of all times says "All men are created equal. Some work harder in pre-season." Life is your pre-season. If you want something than stop talking about it. Stop thinking about it. Go out and get it.

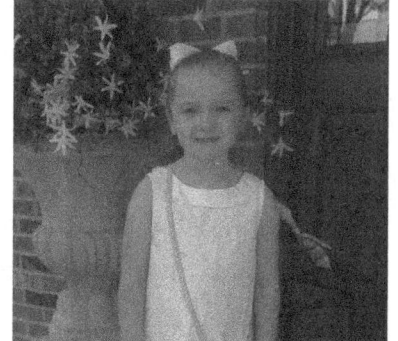

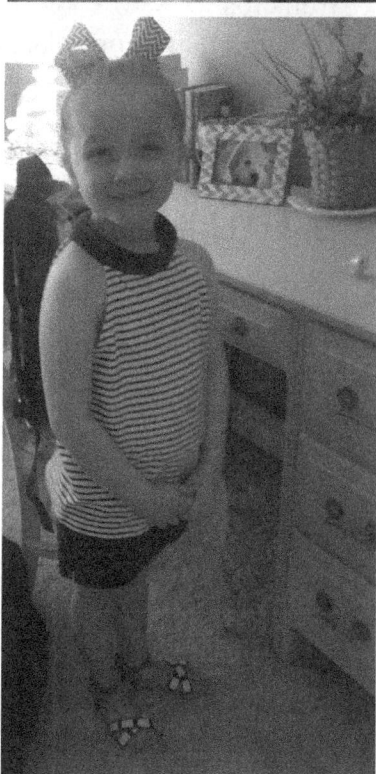

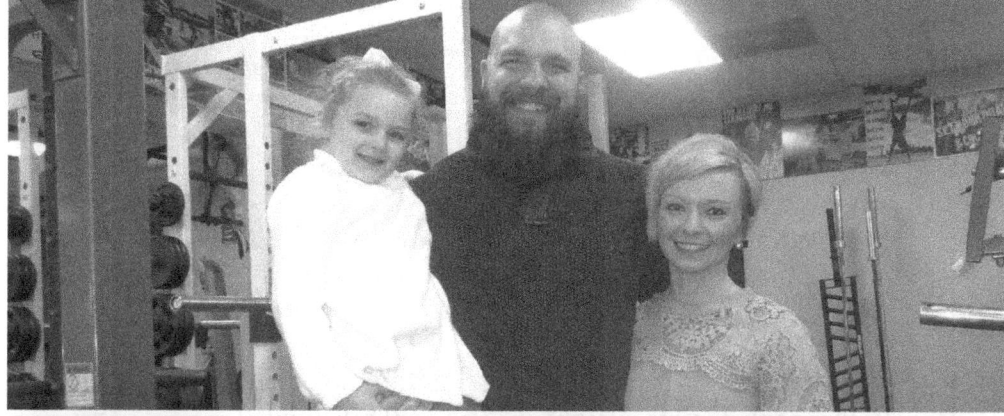

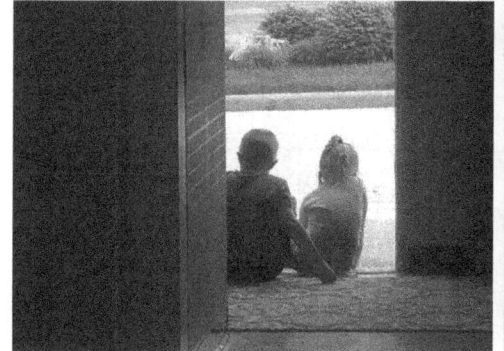

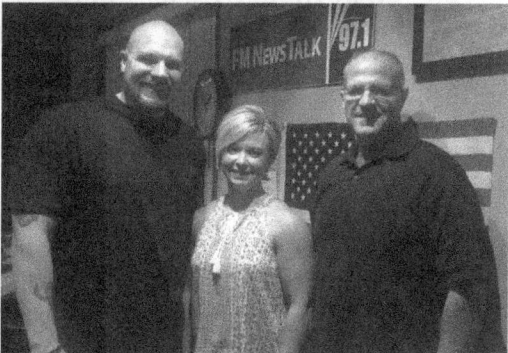

Workouts that explain my style of training:

Workout 1: *Shoulders*
4 sets
10 reps

1. Seated knuckle out shoulder press
   Standing db lateral raise
   Standing db chicken wing
   100 jump ropes

2. Seated Arnold press
   Standing Bent-over rear delt fly thumbs out
   Iron cross
   100 alternating rope slams

3. Cable upright row
   Barbell push press
   Bent-over V-ups
   40 shoulder jack with dumb bells

Workout 2: *Back*
10 reps
4 sets

1. Wide pull ups
   Wide lat pull down
   Wide seated cable row
   1 min rower

2. Close grip pull ups
   Seated cable row close grip
   Seated close grip pull down
   1 min versa climber

3. Cable high row standing
   Reverse pec deck
   Back Ext with db high row
   100 rope slams

Workout 3: *Arms*
4 sets
20 reps

1. Cable double bicep curl
   Db hammer curl
   Bench dips
   20 crunches

2. Cable straight bar extensions
   Overhead cable straight bar extensions
   V bar curls
   20 knee ups hanging

3. Curl Machine
   Db reverse grip curl
   Weighted dip machine
   40 torso twists with weight

Workout 4: *Legs*
4 sets

1. Leg press narrow feet
   20 toes over
   20 toes at top
   20 partial pulses mid point on pad
   2 high push low push on sled

2. Reverse hack squat
   10 feet narrow
   10 feet wide
   20 Db plia squats
   10 Step ups
   1 minute sprint on a 5 incline

3. 10 Db Romanian deadlift
   10 single leg ham curls
   10 single leg press downs (pull up machine)
   1 min sprint on stairs

4. 20 walking weighted lunges
   20 walking weighted crossover lunges
   100 high knees

Workout 5: *Chest*
4 sets
10 reps

1. Incline Smith bench press
   20 pushups
   20 ball slams

2. Db decline press
   20 pushups
   15 tire flips

3. Hammer Strength Chest Press
   20 push ups
   20/20 sledgehammer

Chest cont'd

4. Cable mid point fly
   20 push ups
   100 jump ropes

Workout 6: *Interval Cardio*
4 sets

1. 100 alternating rope slams
   10 burpees with dumbbells
   20 crunches with a punch at the top

2. 4 minutes of running on 5 incline
   4 minutes backwards on stairs
   2 minutes on rower

3. 100 hanging knees
   100 overhead crunches
   Only one set of this to finish.

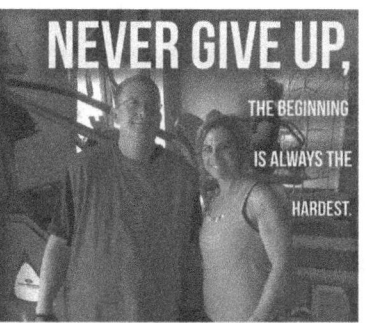
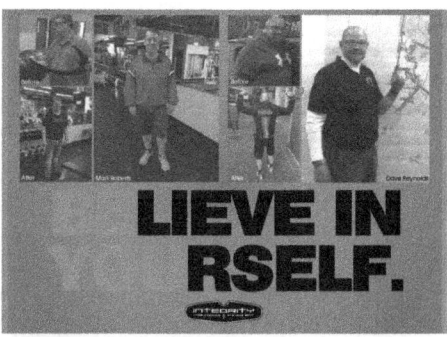
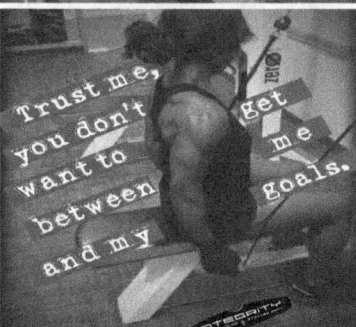
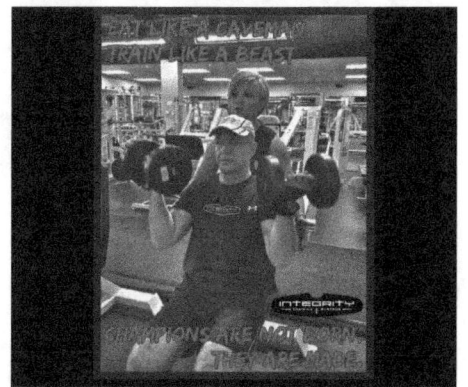
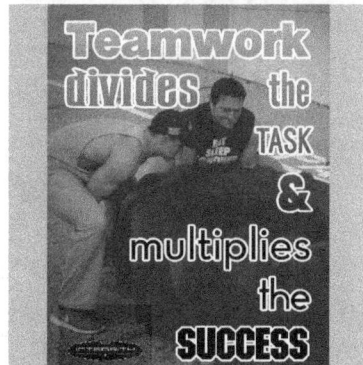
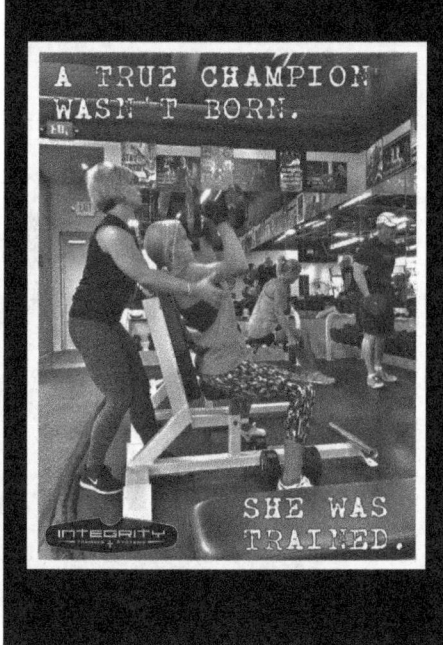
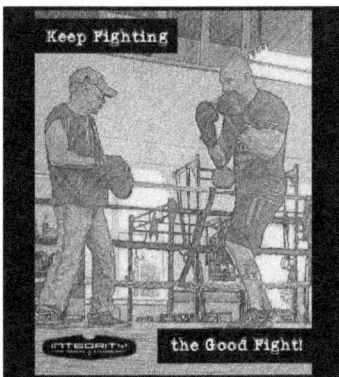
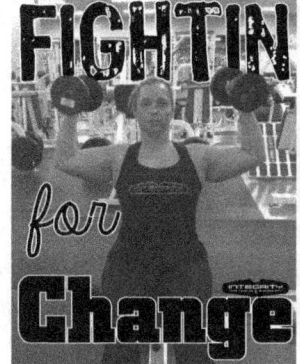
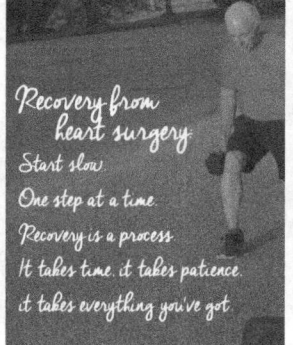

My favorite quotes:

- You are what you do, not what you say you'll do.

- Dead people receive more flowers than the living ones because regret is stronger than gratitude. — Anne Frank

- I can do all things through Christ who strengthens me. Philippians 4:13

- "Complaining about a problem without posing a solution is called whining." —Teddy Roosevelt

- Every day is a fresh start.

- I already know what giving up feels like. I want to see what happens if I don't. — Neila Rey

- some of my best friends never say a word to me

- She is clothed in strength and dignity and she laughs without fear of the future

- >> Enjoy the little things <<

- You are your only Limit.

- Someone once told me not to bite off more than I could chew. I said I'd rather choke on greatness than nibble on mediocrity.

The Armor of God

10 Finally, be strong in the Lord and in his mighty power. **11** Put on the full armor of God, so that you can take your stand against the devil's schemes. **12** For our struggle is not against flesh and blood, but against the rulers, against the authorities, against the powers of this dark world and against the spiritual forces of evil in the heavenly realms. **13** Therefore put on the full armor of God, so that when the day of evil comes, you may be able to stand your ground, and after you have done everything, to stand. **14** Stand firm then, with the belt of truth buckled around your waist, with the breastplate of righteousness in place, **15** and with your feet fitted with the readiness that comes from the gospel of peace. **16** In addition to all this, take up the shield of faith, with which you can extinguish all the flaming arrows of the evil one. **17** Take the helmet of salvation and the sword of the Spirit, which is the word of God.

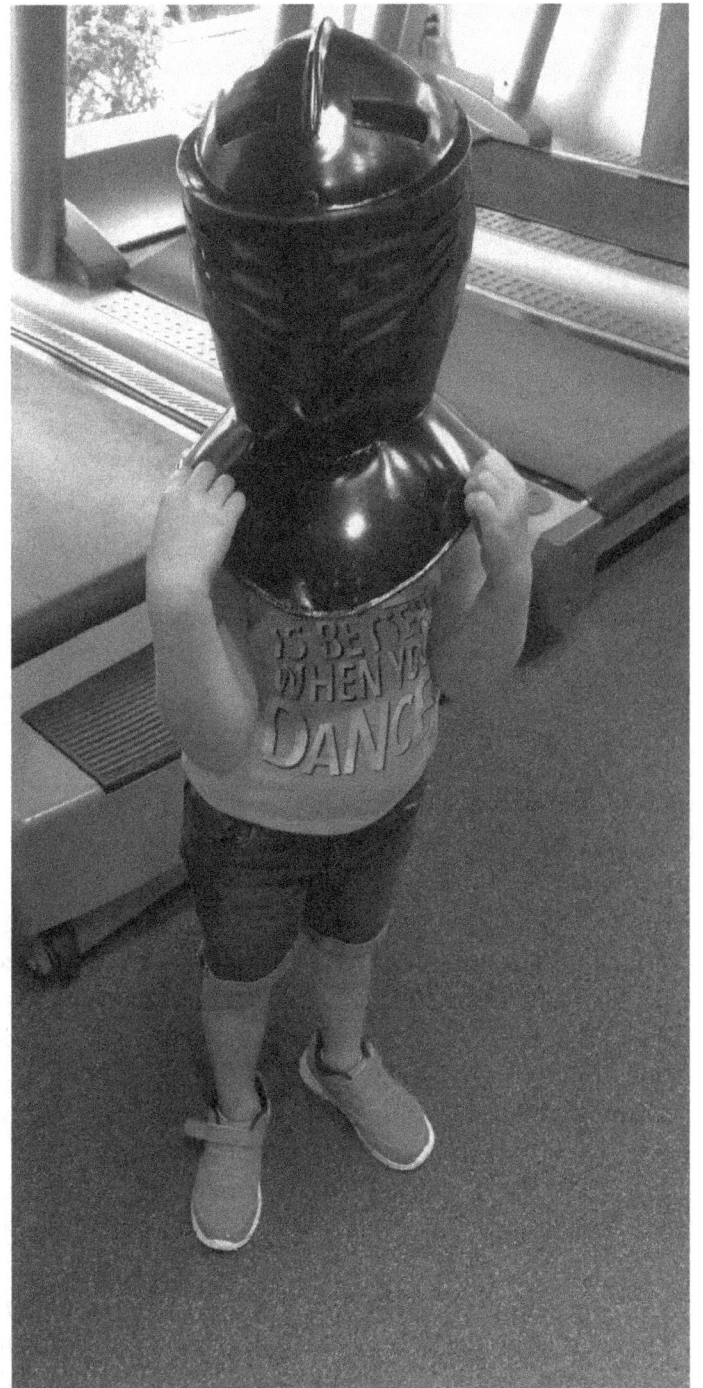

Client Testimony:
-Casey Devine

Hi my name is Casey Devine. Throughout high school I was into all types of athletics, but primarily played competitive tennis. Although, I was very successful in tennis, one thing holding me back was my health such as migraines, seizers, depression, and anxiety. As most people would I sought out help from my primary doctor. I began taking multiple medications for all of my health problems I was experiencing along with seeing specialist for migraines. I cannot count how many medications I tried throughout the process. Even being on medication I still had the same problems also with side affects. Not one doctor ever talked to me about nutrition, so I ate basically whatever I wanted and whenever I wanted. Fast food was a daily choice, not to mention I consumed at least 32oz of diet coke a day. I began to feel as though I just needed to learn to live with all the health problems. Two years after graduating high school I became pregnant with my daughter Ivanna. Throughout the pregnancy I stopped taking all medications and was advised to watch my sodium intake and stop drinking soda due to severe swelling. I noticed during my pregnancy I didn't get one single migraine or seizure. After having Ivanna I slowly merged back into a bad food habit and even more soda than before. I woke up with a headache every morning, I was always tired, and very depressed. I began missing work once a month around my cycle from migraines and seizers again which lead to more medication again..... I struggled with this for about 3 years until I was fed up and decided to seek other options.

I began working out more often and met new friends there along the way. Nutrition is a common subject talked about at gyms and I began researching on my own. I started making healthier options and slowly stopped taking my medicines. Meanwhile my mother was seeing Debbie for nutrition counseling and recommended I go see her because she and was able to get off her blood pressure medication. I began training with Debbie every week and slowly starting learning how food and exercise can benefit your health. As time went on I realized that all the preservatives and added hormones in the food I was eating was elevating my hormones and causing all these issues. I am proud to say as of today I am not taking any medications and have been migraine/seizure free for about 2 years. I love all the knowledge I have learned though training with Debbie so much that I decided to get my Nasm certification. During the Nasm process I started to understand what Debbie preached at me for the last year. She always told me about my muscle imbalances and how I needed to work on strengthening my back to help my posture. I finally listened and feel stronger during all of my workouts and see a huge difference in my posture. I now see working out just as normal as brushing your teeth every morning and meal prepping became a Monday ritual not only for me, but my family as well. I don't see this as a fad or a diet I see the way we live as a lifestyle. Like most people, I have cravings. I struggle with sugar in particular and have learned how serious and close to a drug it really is and how addicting it is to me. Knowing I surround myself with people at Integrity with the same struggles, mindset and goals such as myself has helped keep me on track tremendously. The feeling I get during my workouts now after re-balancing my body and eating consistently clean is indescribable. I have learned my body is a temple and I will continue to cherish it.

One of my favorite quotes is,
" Let food be thy medicine and medicine be thy food"- Hippocrates

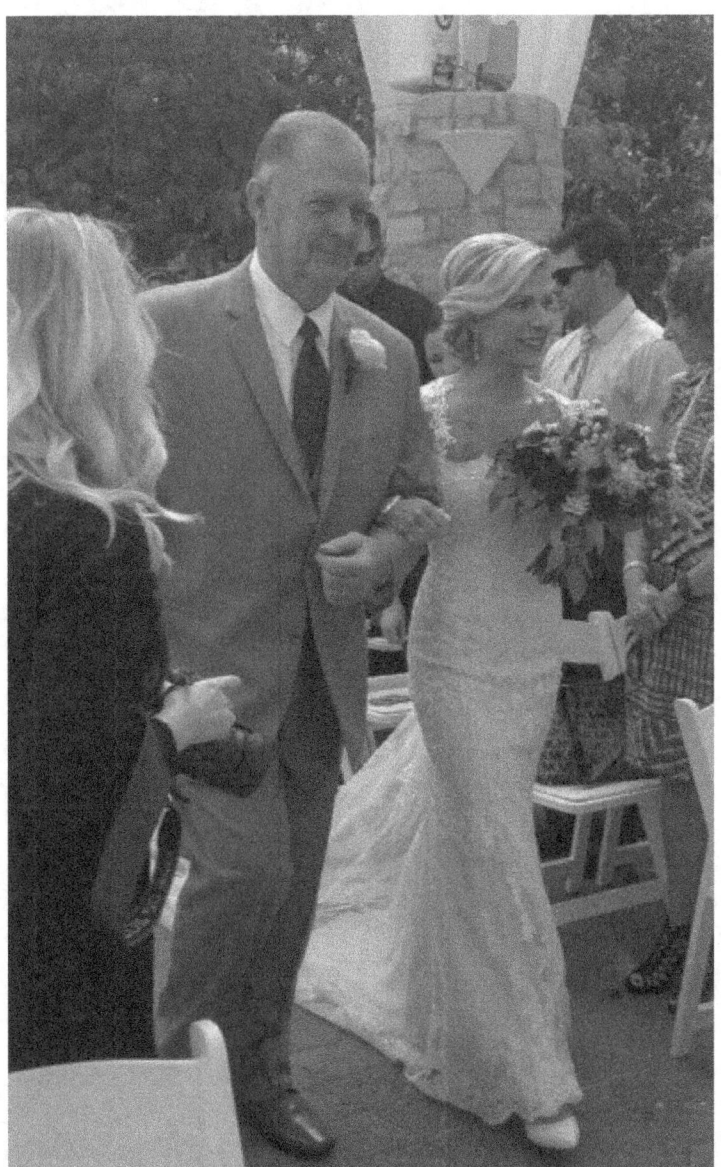
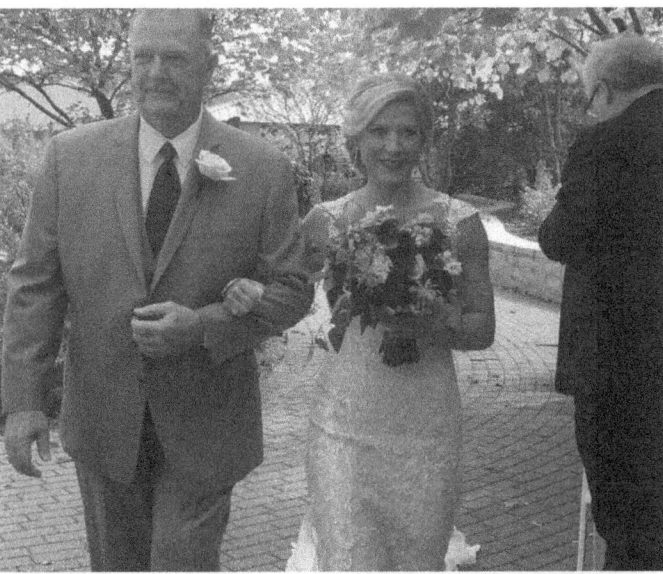
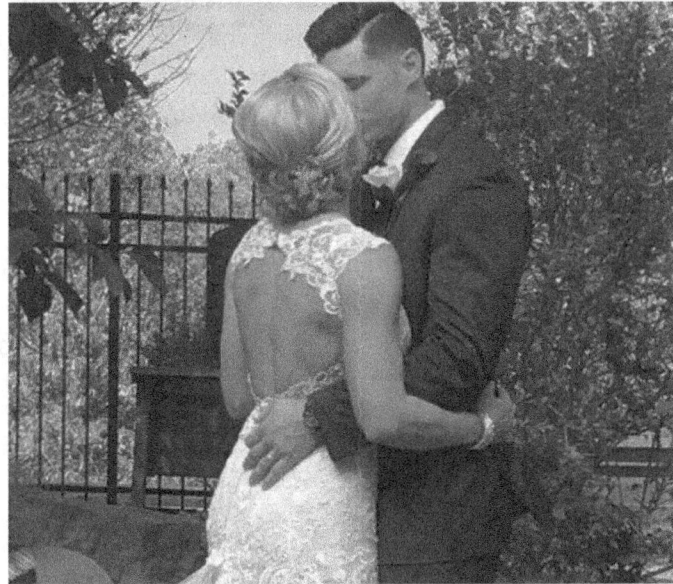

Client Testimony:
-Stacy Hess

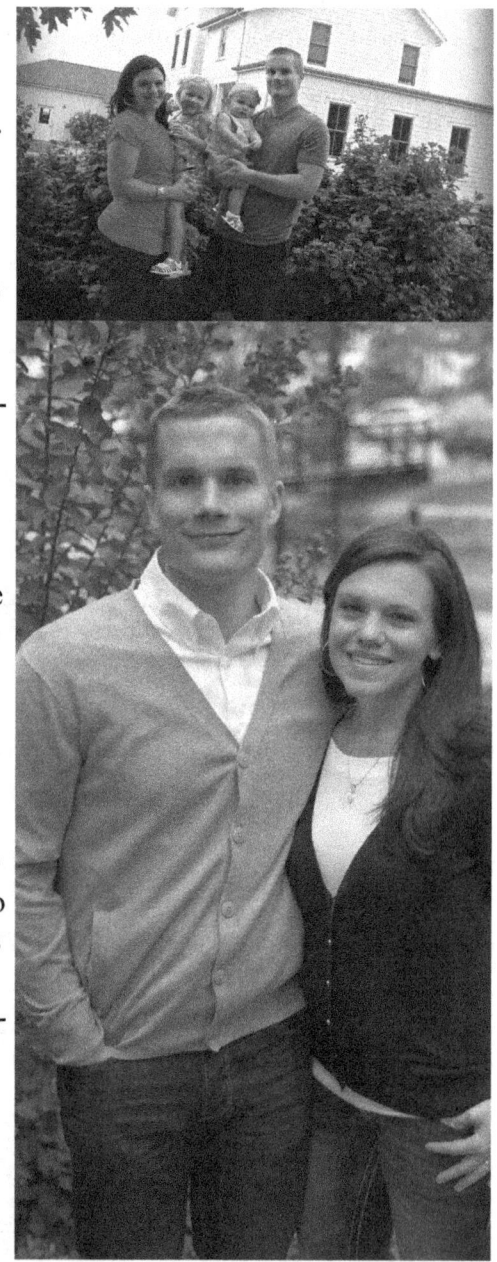

We were referred to Debbie Portell for help with weight loss in the summer of 2013. After seeing the results several of our friends experienced after working with her, we decided to do our first "joint" weight loss effort as a couple. After having 2 beautiful babies within just over 2 years, our health had taken the back-burner. Debbie took the time to educate us instead of simply prescribing a meal plan. She learned about our goals and then set the foundation for living a healthy, clean way of eating. The understanding of the science behind her advice was life-changing. We quickly learned what to eliminate and what to add to our diets, and saw immediate results. The weight loss was exciting, as I had tried every gimmick and plan in the book with no results. Debbie's advice showed us both quick results on the scale, but amazingly in other areas too. I had not been able to run for years, my joints hurt too much; but once the inflammation had declined I could run without pain. I completed a 10k one year after starting to work with Debbie. We were in better moods, saw increased productivity at work, decrease in sickness and seasonal allergies, and improved health screenings. We were genuinely enjoying our new lifestyle. It came to the point where we preferred to eat clean versus the fried foods we used to enjoy. Most importantly, we realized what a difference we could make for our daughters health. They learned early that "Miss Debbie" helps our family eat healthy so we can live better lives.

After a few years, the weight started slowly creeping back on and poor old habits were taking over. We knew exactly what would work, and so we re-connected with Debbie. She continuously and tirelessly supports our family. Her dedication and loyalty and consistency has made an extreme difference in the life of our family and so many friends. Learning the foundation and tools behind clean eating has been life changing. We are so ever thankful.

Client Testimony:
-The Scharf Family

-Sandi Scharf

I fortunately met Debbie because of my husband's search for help for his chronic body pain and to help our sons remain injury free and competitive in their sports endeavors. He scheduled an appointment for our family to meet with her to discuss exercise and nutrition advice. I went into the meeting thinking that I was there primarily to support my family because I do most of the shopping and food preparation.

 Debbie focused on each of us as individuals and she helped me tremendously with my chronic digestive issues. She listened carefully to what I was eating and drinking and to my exercise routine. She made recommendations for nutritional changes and increased water intake and with her advice I no longer have the digestive issues I had for 30 years of my life! She was able to get me to understand that what I was eating was causing my issues and that I did not need prescriptions or surgery to help myself. Since following Debbie's recommendations, I have felt more energetic, and I am able think more clearly, have been able to maintain a healthy weight, and have been following a regular exercise routine including lifting weights and jogging at age 55!

Even long after out meetings, Debbie has so graciously remained available to answer any of our questions regarding making good food choices, recipe ingredient substitutions and exercise. Debbie thank you so much for helping us !!!

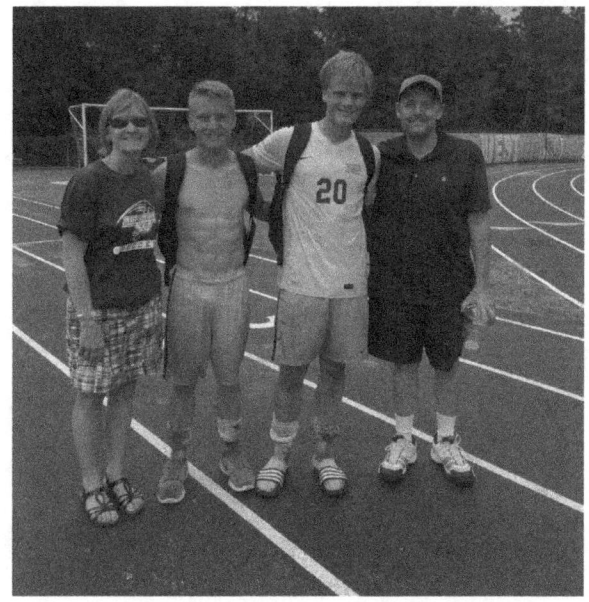

Client Testimony:
-The Scharf Family

-John Scharf

September 1, 2015, 202 pounds, July 1, 2016, weight has leveled out at 155 pounds! C-Reactive Protein, inflammatory marker was elevated at around 6.5 for many years and now is at 2.2, well within the normal range! Although my diet was not horrible relative to the standard American diet, Debbie worked with me as to my specific needs and brought me light years ahead in greatly reducing inflammation and weight as well as increasing energy and mental clarity.

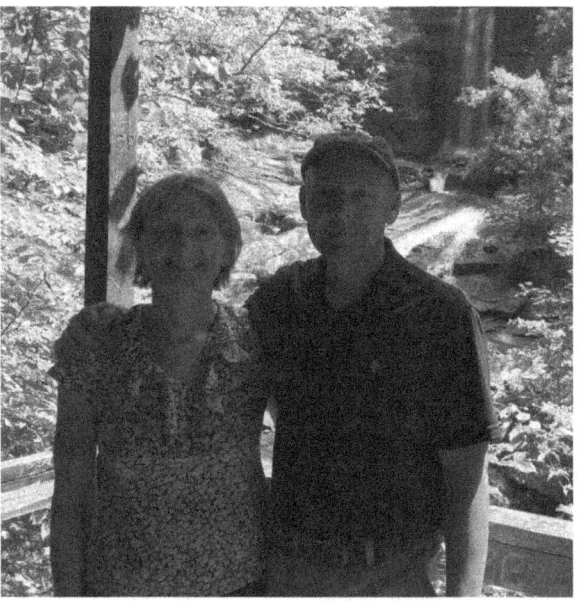

I have been training with integrity fitness and making strong progress physically and structurally as well. This has all been very helpful for me in dealing with inflammatory issues and neck, back and lower body structural issues which are quite intense. The unending time and caringness that Debbie has put in for me and my family has been a blessing and has been positive for us as to each our individual lifestyle needs.

We look forward to working with Debbie for years to come and I know that the hard work she puts forth to share her knowledge and experience will bring about a healthy and happier future for us as well as many others.

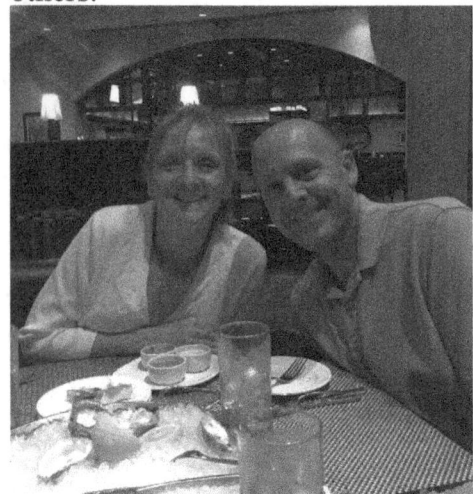

Client Testimony:
-The Scharf Family

-Michael Scharf

Since the start of working with Debbie at Integrity Fitness, I have noticed great improvement in my overall performance as an athlete. I am a collegiate soccer player so the physical strain put on my body year round can be quite high. I am on the field six to seven days a week and do weight lifting on top of that so I knew nutrition would be the key to improving as a player.

Before working with Debbie, I had experienced issues with inflammation and injuries; I would experience muscle strains, tendinitis, and joint pain. These injuries held back my development as a player and at times kept me sidelined from the game altogether. When my family decided to begin working with Integrity Fitness I hoped that a change in nutrition would help me alleviate some of these issues.

Debbie was able to show me how to truly target what foods my body needed (or didn't need) and how the foods I ate would affect my body's inflammatory process, recovery ability, and overall output on the field as well as in the weight room. I have since seen dramatic improvement in my ability to quickly recover from wear and tear on a daily basis. Injuries have been minimal if any; inflammation is better dealt with and injuries are prevented. I have been able to play many more minutes than my teammates without injury and with less fatigue. I have also been able to create a good source of energy for games through pregame meals that Debbie has helped me plan which has helped me maintain more consistent performances over the course of my season.

I will definitely take the nutrition principles I have learned from Integrity Fitness forward with me throughout my playing career as I push to reach higher and higher levels, as well as further in my life after my competitive playing days are over. My change in nutrition has really opened my eyes to the power of food and the role it can play for athletes looking to improve their game.

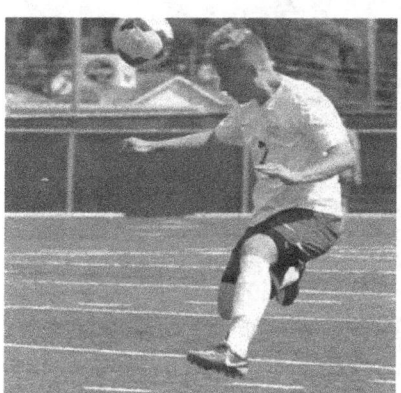

Client Testimony:
-The Scharf Family

-Matthew Scharf

As an 18 year old collegiate soccer player, I was able to lose ten pounds and sustain a lean, healthy weight with Debbie's advice and passion for nutrition. This difference helped my stay fit, kept me from getting injuries and allowed my body to recover quickly when playing at a high level of soccer. Every time my family and I visited in order to get advice from Debbie, she showed so much devotion to helping us live a healthier life that it truly changed the way we thought about nutrition and exercise. By altering our attitudes and understanding of the things we put in our body everyday and how we train our body, Debbie was able to help change my family's life for the positive!

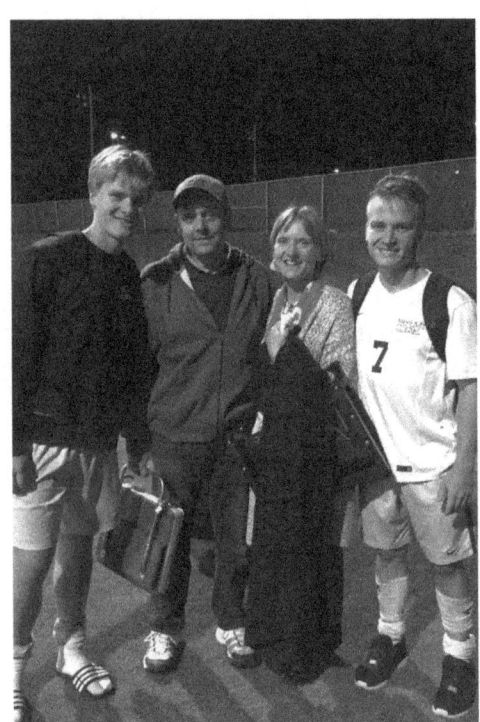
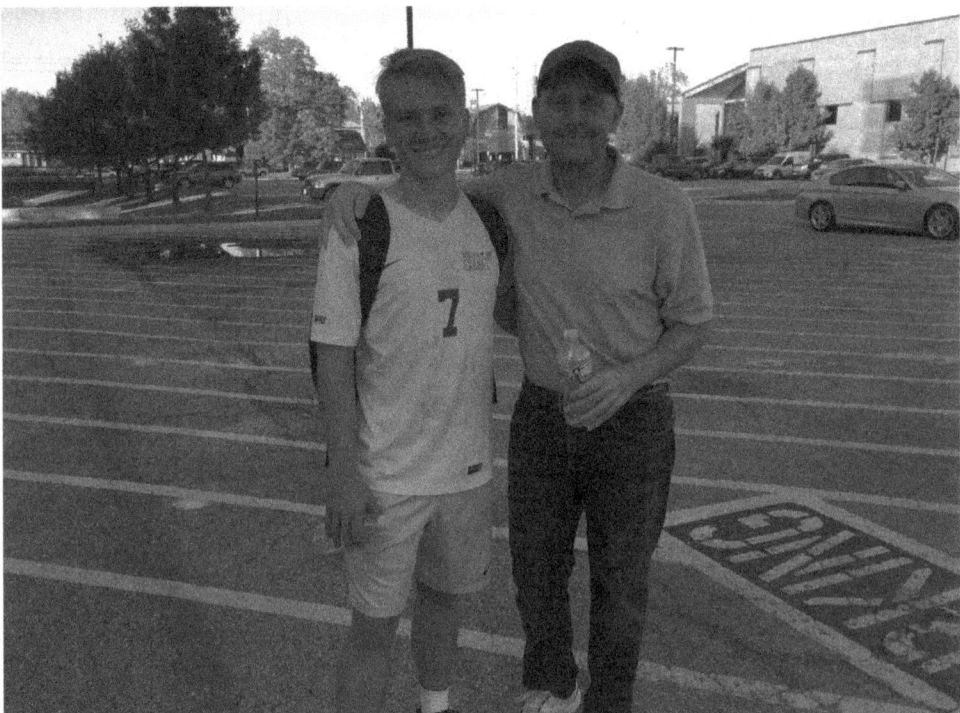

Client Testimony:
-Randy Halstead

With a consistently hectic schedule at work and at home, I have difficulty finding time to focus on my own personal well-being. This has led to an increase in health-related issues over the past twenty years, for both me and my wife. Seeking help from medical doctors has never produced any real solutions, as they simply played the blame game or prescribed pills. But while the doctors gave up, my son didn't. Ryan led us to Integrity Training Systems. Debbie Portell understood the struggles of diabetes, high blood pressure, and thyroid disease. She didn't focus on blaming past decisions, but led through education, encouragement, and support. Today, I am healthier and more active. I am in better control of what I eat to fuel my body and more knowledgeable about how to perform the physical exercise my body requires. My weight is now maintained, and I have reduced or eliminated several of my medications. I'm proud to say my wife and daughter have been equally successful through Debbie's guidance. I am still challenged by my hectic schedule to make the best choices. Sometimes I don't. But I do know that Debbie will be there to help get me back on the right path.

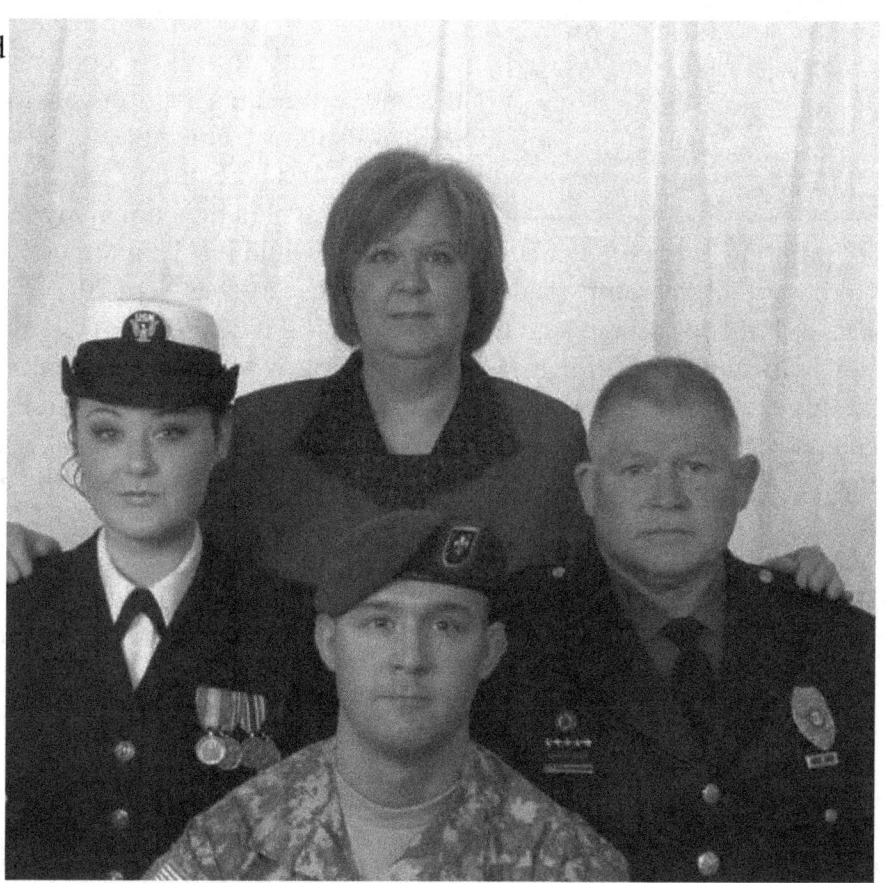

The Road to Recovery
Bill & Barb Clark; Father & Mother

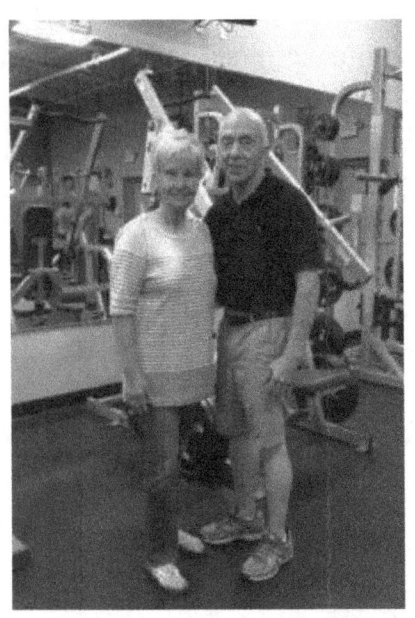

August 31, 2010 I suffered a heart attack. My heart stopped. I was with Barb at Gold's gym on highway K. Two young employees, Gerald and Stephanie, had just been trained on the defibrillator 2 weeks before. They shocked me back to life. The paramedics that showed up while taking me to the hospital, Barb was riding along, had to shock me with the defibrillator again. I was taken to St Peters Barnes Emergency and moved to ICU. I was unconscious for 14 days. In an induced coma packed in ice. God Bless the staff in the ICU at St Peters Barnes. When I came out of the coma I didn't remember any of it. Barb explained what had happen but I did not fully understand. Our insurance would not pay for surgery at St Peters Barnes. I was moved by ambulance to St Josephs, St Charles. I love the staff there. The nurses that were on duty and all the doctors that saw me daily.

The same paramedics that took me to St Peters Barnes moved me to St Josephs. I slightly remember it. It was not a ride I enjoyed. I think I wondered why I was here. I don't remember anything. I remember waking up from surgery with a tube down my throat. The nurse was talking to me. I kept pointing at the tube. She assured me it would just be a minute. The next thing I remember was being in a room with my family and nurses. The surgery was Sept 20.

I had an infection which kept me in the hospital much longer than normal. The nurses and staff were great. They helped me get through each shift. Along with my family. Barb was there every day along with Bob and Roger Semsch. Debbie and Kim were there often helping Mom with what they could. Their smiles and encouragement kept me going. Thank them all. I love them for it. I was weak and surprised by it. I remember standing in front of a mirror and wrapping my right hand around my left arm. I had lost weight; muscle and fat. The nurses would have me go for walks. They encouraged me. Tried to make me feel good. Each day was a milestone. Walking down the hall and back. As often as I wanted. At first only a few times. Then maybe once an hour. The doctors came every day. I loved seeing them. They and many others saved my life. I felt strongly about that and still do. I went home Oct 6. Seemed like I had been there forever. God Bless you all.

The Journey:

Just getting home didn't make everything alright. Now became the recovery back. I was weak. Very weak. We lived in a 2 story home. In the hospital they would walk me up 19 stair steps; check my heart rate and oxygen and then walk me back down and check be again. Once a day they would do that. That was to prepare me for the stairs at home. I knew I could walk up them. The first few months I stayed at the ground level except for going up to shower each day. Started physical therapy at Lake St Louis St Josephs. Started with 3 lb. dumbbells. 6 weeks later I moved to cardiac rehab. I was up to 5 lbs, but they moved me back to 3 lbs. Moved up each week. Started slow and worked up. Treadmill, bike, shoulder cardio machine and light weights. After 8 weeks I moved to the other side. Same exercises but I was in control. No more sensors tracking my heart. They check you when you came in and when you were done before you could leave. They watched over me and got me back. Just remember you will recover. It just takes time. That was the best advice my brother David gave me when I came out of the hospital. That comment stuck with me and always helped me to keep going. Watch what you eat and do the exercises. After 2 years Barb let me move to a real gym. She was scared and worried about me (and still does). It is not something you get over. I wore a heart monitor for several months. Started slow. Light weights 2 days a week. Cardio 3 days a week. Rotating workouts. I would do 8-10 reps 1st week. 12-15 reps the 2nd week. When I reached 18 reps and 2 sets I would move up in weight after 2 or 3 weeks of 18. I would repeat the process 8-10 reps. I have reached a maintenance level now. Gone from 3 lb. to 30 lb. dumbbells. 3 days of cardio and 2 days of weights. Full body on the weights except for chest. Because of surgery the Doctor doesn't want me working chest. It's a good workout keeping me in shape. 6 years of it. Allows me to do the things I did 15-20 years ago. Exercise and nutrition does that. Get started now. Start slow and you will get there. At some point you get caught up in it and want more. You will like how you feel. The cardio has gone from 10-15 min treadmill at 1.5-2.5 to 47 min at 3.6, 3.7, and 3.8 at 10 min increments. For 30 min with an incline of 5.0 walking. Then, not stopping, 1 mile running at 10:45 min/mile; then ½ mile at 10:00 min/mile finishing a 9:00 min/mile for 10-20 sec sprint.

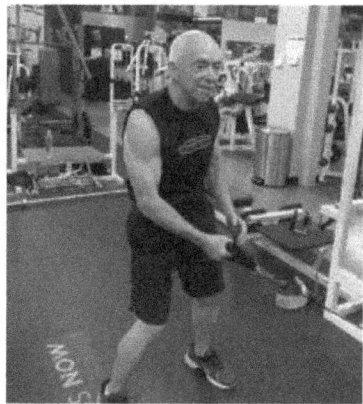
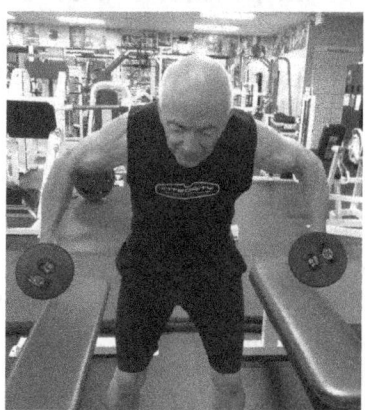
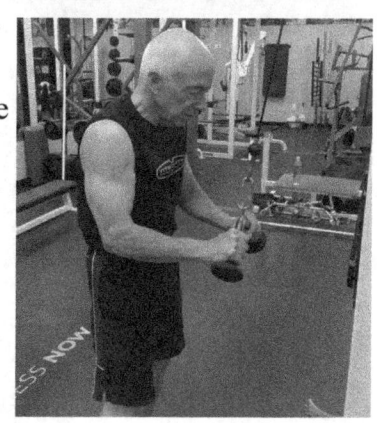

What is your philosophy on nutrition?

Good clean food changes our life. You can still eat well at each meal and stay healthy. When I came home from the hospital Debbie showed up on Sunday with a week's worth of food and my meal plan. She had purchased and cooked it all. After a month or so Barb would prepare all the meals on Sunday allowing Deb to take Sunday off from us. She would still come out, but we would buy the food and cook it on Sundays. It is all great food. Some of it so good you can't stop fixing it. For 6 years I have maintained my weight of 150 lb. Not moving above 150 more than 2 lb. or less. I feel what I have to eat tastes great, I love to eat it and have great results.

I continue to receive great results at the Doctor's visits. I get blood work every 6 months. My cholesterol stays at 131-136 overall. Triglycerides are low averaging 70s. HDL is great to me. Been in 60+ for 6 years. And LDL stays at 70s.

My Digestion is great as well. Before my heart attack I kept Tums, Rolaids and Pepcid AC in my desk at work. I have not had indigestion once in 6 years. It's the clean food. My gut is balanced.

My energy level is great. I don't get tired or hungry. It surprises me. I find it hard to explain to others. I can remember in the past if I did something for a long duration of time I would get tired. At the end of a wok out now I am not tired. I could do more but because of time I don't. At the end of the day I might be sleepy but I am not tired. I would play 2 – 36 hole golf tournaments each year. By the 27 hole you are ready to stop. The ones I play now I finish 36 and feel great and my friends are done in. Educate yourself on food. No regrets.

The message is that you can recover from a heart attack. It takes time and effort. Take it slow. Exercise and clean food. It is easier to prevent a heart attack then recover from on. Start now.

The Power of Prayer: God works miracles and I feel I am one. For those who prayed for me daily and those who came and laid hands on me and prayed I thank you. God blesses you every day in every way!!!
Bill & Barb

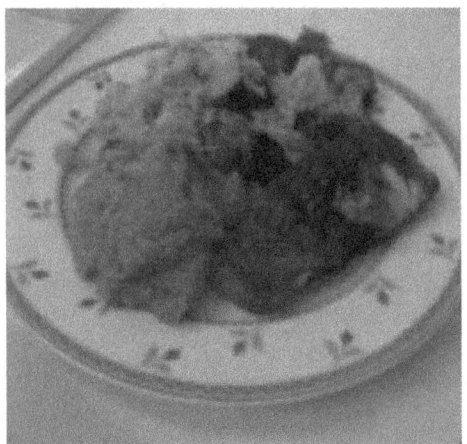
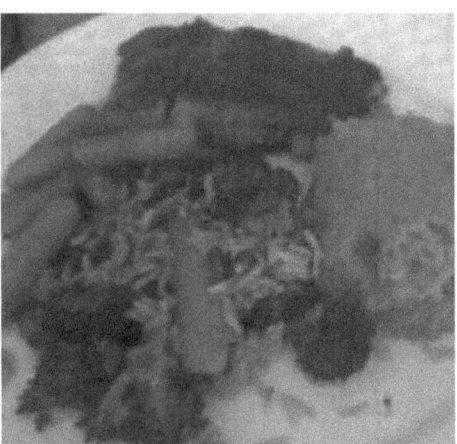
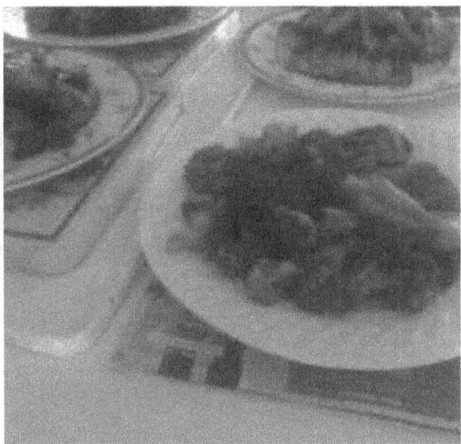

What made you a trainer?
-John Morris

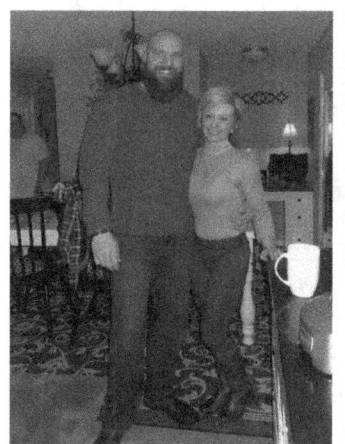

God made me a trainer. I have always wanted to help people my entire life. As a young child I was very sickly and told my parents I wanted to be a doctor so I could help people feel better.

While I was in college I decided to go into law enforcement, again with the belief that I could make the world a better place. The Lord showed me this was not my calling. Unfortunately I was so hard headed it required poor health and a heart attack to do so.

What inspires you?

You do. No not the one who asked the question but you reading this. Whatever your reason is, it has to do with you wanting to be better. I wake up everyday to help you with that. If I can help one person go through the dramatic life change that I did, then I can call my life successful.

What are your strengths?

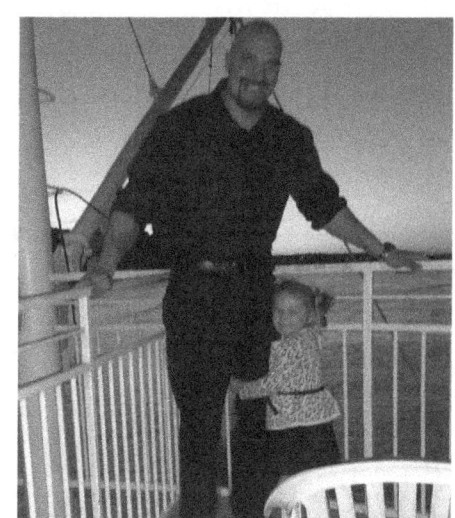

My failures are my strengths. When a bone breaks, it grows back stronger. My mind, body and spirit have been broken and what did not kill me has made me stronger. I am sympathetic and empathetic to the struggles of life but driven to help those struggling to persevere.

Weaknesses?

Where do I even start on this? First off I am just as human as you and will fall on some of the same trials of life. My mind is weak and requires daily motivation to keep strong. So when you have a day where you just "aren't feeling it" know that I can relate, but like me, you can push through it.

What has your focus? What are your goals?

My focus is on growing Integrity so that it can touch as many lives as possible. I want to know when I die that my work helped change as many lives as possible.

What is your philosophy on nutrition?

Nutrition is everything Originally working with Integrity Training Systems as a client my only goal was to lose 100 pounds. I did that. There is no way I could have done with without proper nutrition. Beyond the physical aspects of proper nutrition there is also the less talked about neurological aspects. I suffer from multiple mental disorders such as depression, anxiety and even bi-polar. When I lock my food down, and eat what I am supposed to, these symptoms dissipate without the use of medication.

What do you eat and why?

I stick to whole foods. I also try to avoid high amounts of complex carbohydrates, sugars and dairy because they seem to be the primary triggers for the neurological issues I spoke of earlier.

Do you take supplements?

I do not. I have taken things like glutamine or branch chain amino acids in the past but usually find myself forgetting to take them.

What is your workout schedule & why?

I like to break my workouts into individual major muscle groups. An example would be:

Monday: *Legs*
Tuesday: *Chest*
Wednesday: *Back*
Thursday: *Shoulders*
Friday: *Legs*
Saturday: *Rest*
Sunday: *Rest*

I will work the respective minor muscles such as triceps on chest day and biceps on back day. Workouts average between 1 and 2 hours.

I do this because I really like to exercise the specific muscle grouping and force my body to focus specifically on it during the recovery phase.

What is your definition of passion? Heart? Success?

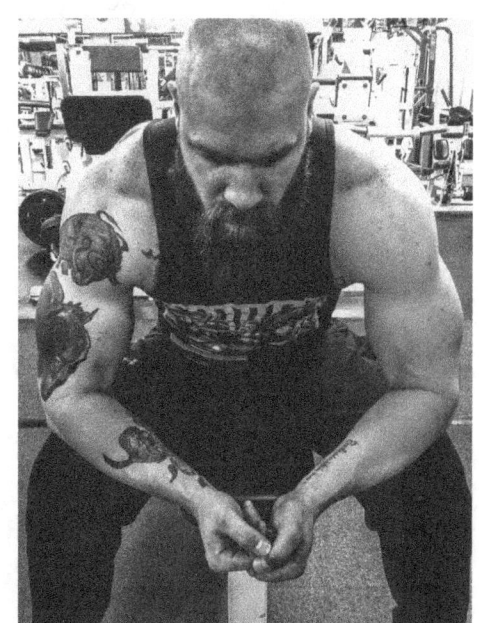

Passion is a strong and barely controllable emotion. I believe it's impossible to hide true passion. It is seen when someone shows up every day and leaves everything they have in what they do.

Heart is having the courage to pursue the unknown. You don't know if you can eat right and exercise? You messed up once when you tried? Did you try again?

Success is going after your passion no matter what it takes to achieve it. You will have failures but success is getting up until you get it right. Have the heart to pursue your passion. Heart leads to perseverance. Perseverance leads to success.

How do you stay motivated to make this a lifestyle and not a goal?

My health condition is what makes me stay motivated. Knowing how dramatically my mind, body and spirit are affected by food and exercise keeps me pressing forward.

What does Train to Live mean to you?

Train to live means getting the most out of life by keeping your mind and body sharp. While it is great to lose weight, gain muscle, or change the way you look, the true focus should be ensuring you get to live the life you have been blessed with. My father once told me prior to changing his lifestyle that he "just wanted to be able to walk around the lake" when he went fishing. That is why I do what I do.

My favorite quotes:

"Sweat more in training so that you bleed less in battle"
"Don't stop when you are tired, stop when you are done"
"You only fail when you stop trying"
If it doesn't challenge you it won't change you"

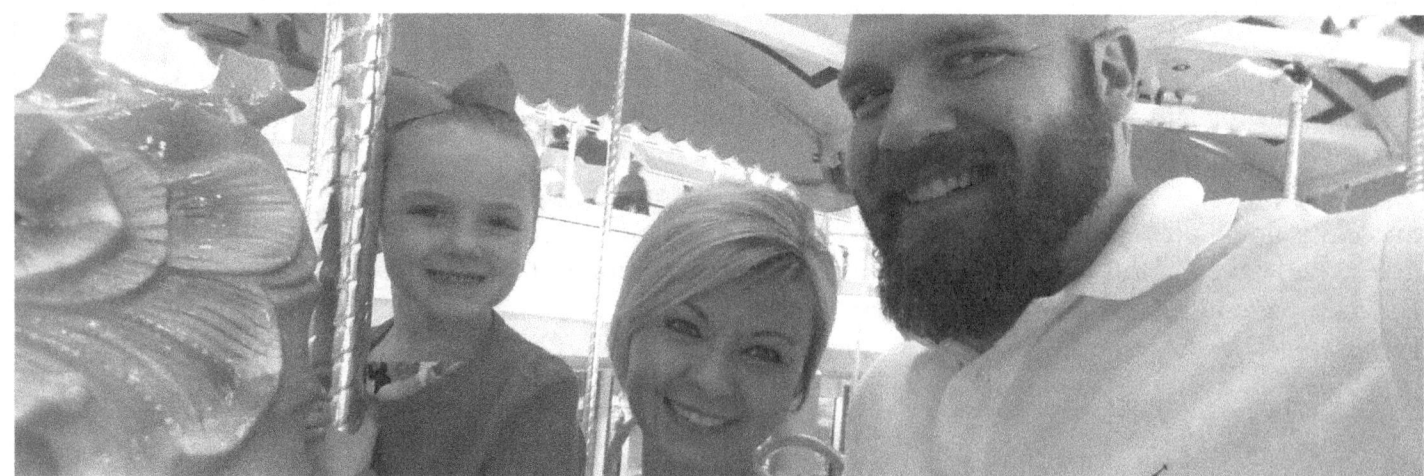

Workouts that explain my style of training:

Workout 1: *Chest*
4 sets, 10 reps

Super set every set of every exercise with 10 pushups

1. Incline bench press (Barbell)
2. Flat bench press (Barbell)
3. Decline bench press (Barbell)
4. Flat bench press (dumbbell)
5. Flat fly (dumbbell)
6. Mid fly (cable or pec dec)

Workout 2: *Back*
4 sets

1. 6 Wide lat pull down
2. 12 Seated close row
3. 20 pull up (wide)
4. Jump rope x100

1. 6 Close lat pull down
2. 12 Seated wide row
3. 20 Close grip pull-ups
4. Slam ball x50

1. 6 Bent over row
2. 12 Bent-over rear fly
3. 20 Underhand pull-up
4. 60 seconds under hand row machine.

Workout 3: *Full Body Strength Training*
4 sets, 10 reps of all

1. Wide-grip lat pull down
2. Close-grip seated row
3. Bent-over rear delt fly
4. Cardio interval 2 mins.

1. Knuckle out press
2. Side lateral
3. Front lateral
4. Cardio interval 2 mins

1. Leg Extension
2. Leg Curl
3. Lunges
4. Cardio interval 2 mins

1. Plank 30 secs
2. Crunch 30 secs
3. Torso twist 30 secs

Workout 4: *Shoulders*
4 sets

1. 6 Dumbbell knuckle out press (seated)
2. 12 side lateral raise
3. 20 Front lateral raise
4. 100 Jump ropes

1. 6 Standing barbell press
2. 12 Front lateral raise
3. 20 Upright row
4. 60 secs Versa climber

1. 6 Cybex shoulder press
2. 12 Side lateral raise
3. 20 Seated side lateral partials
4. 50 Bounce ball slams

Workout 5: *Arms*
4 sets

1. Barbell curl
2. V-bar cable curl
3. Cybex curl machine
4. Free-motion curl

1. Rope tricep pushdown
2. Overhead v-bar tricep extension
3. Close grip press (Smith)
4. Cybex tricep pullover

1. Hammer curl
2. Twist curl
3. Dumbbell overhead extension
4. Dumbbell close press

Workout 5: *Legs*
4 sets

1. Standard leg press x 10
2. Lunges x10 per leg
3. Leg extension x10
4. 60 secs stairs (fast)

1. Toe high leg press x10
2. Reverse lunges (weighted by cable) x10 per leg
3. Leg curl x10
4. 60 secs of stairs (fast)

1. Single leg push down x 10 per leg
2. Seated adductor x10 per leg
3. Glute kickback x10 per leg
4. 60 seconds of stairs (fast)

Why Choose Integrity?

Choose Integrity because you intend to make your health a priority and change your lifestyle. Integrity will be in it for the long haul with you. Both trainers and clients will motivate you and be there for you much like a family. You will always feel welcome and will never be judged. This of course is not even mentioning how qualified the trainers are to get you the results you are looking for.

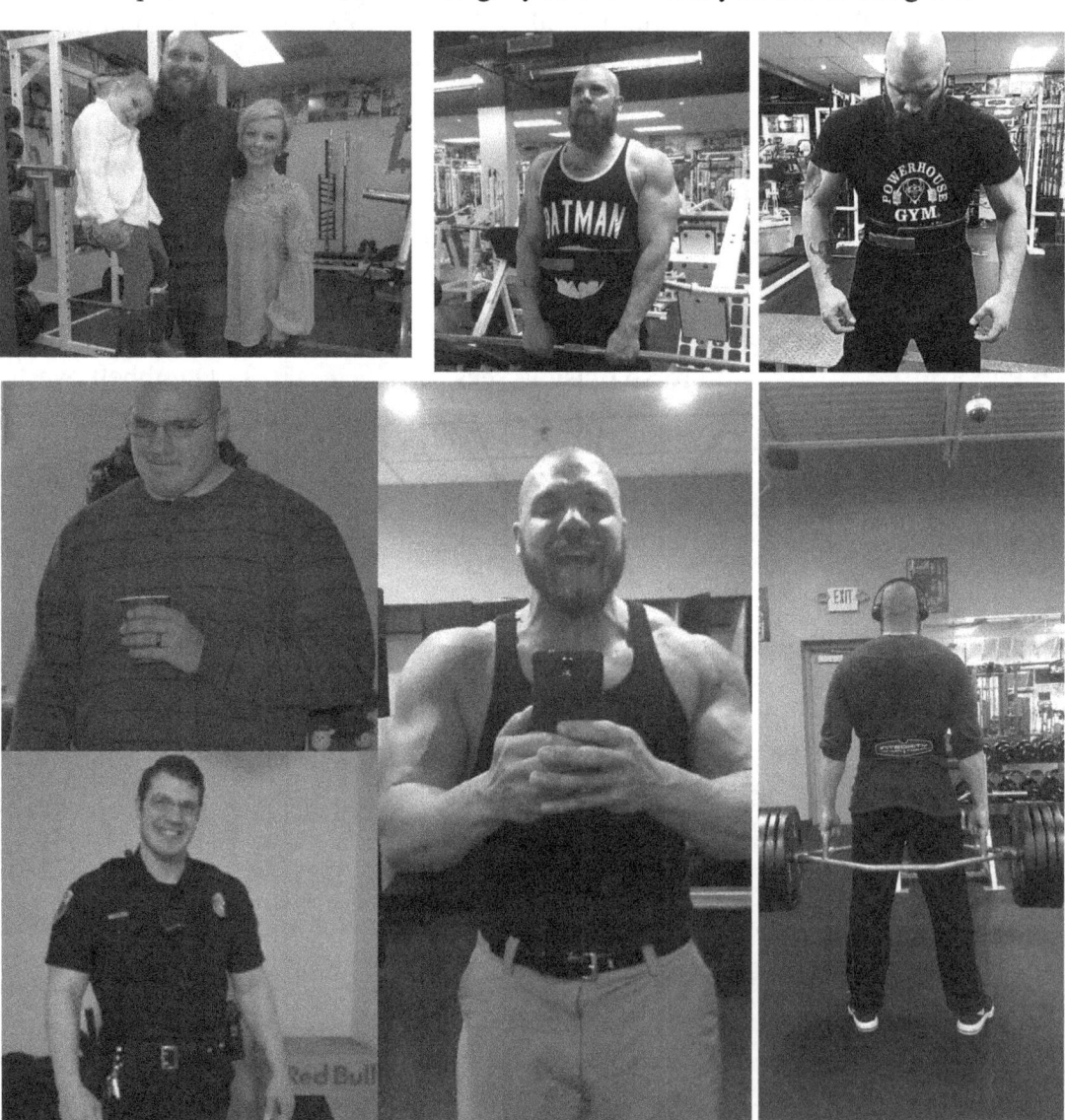

Client Testimony:
-Ryan Halstead

When I first met John and Debbie I had recently gotten out of a bad relationship and was in the worst shape of my life. Through their fitness guidance, motivational personalities, and nutritional plan I was able to completely turn myself around into the best shape of my life, recently joining the Regional SWAT team. Thanks to John and Debbie, my life has improved to a level I had never thought was possible again. Integrity doesn't sell you on gimmicky diets and workout routines, rather solid lifestyle changes and proper form and technique to get the results you desire.

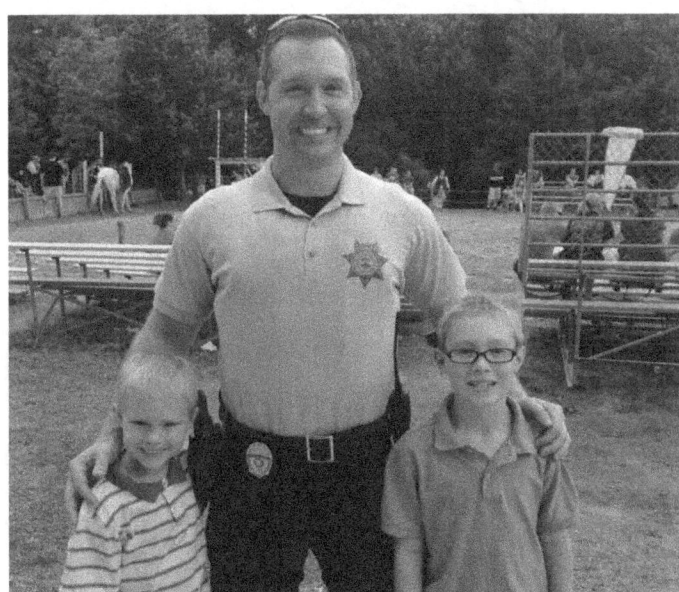

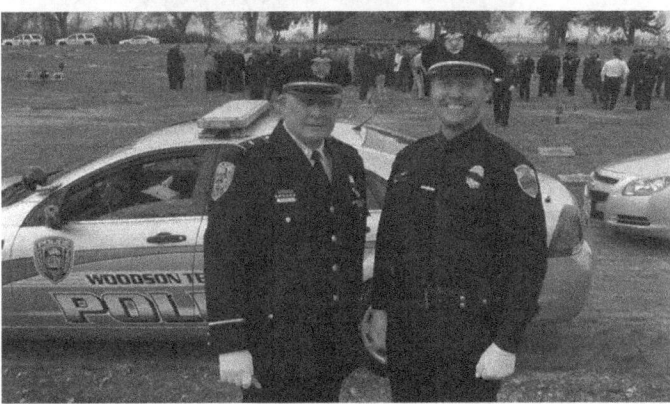

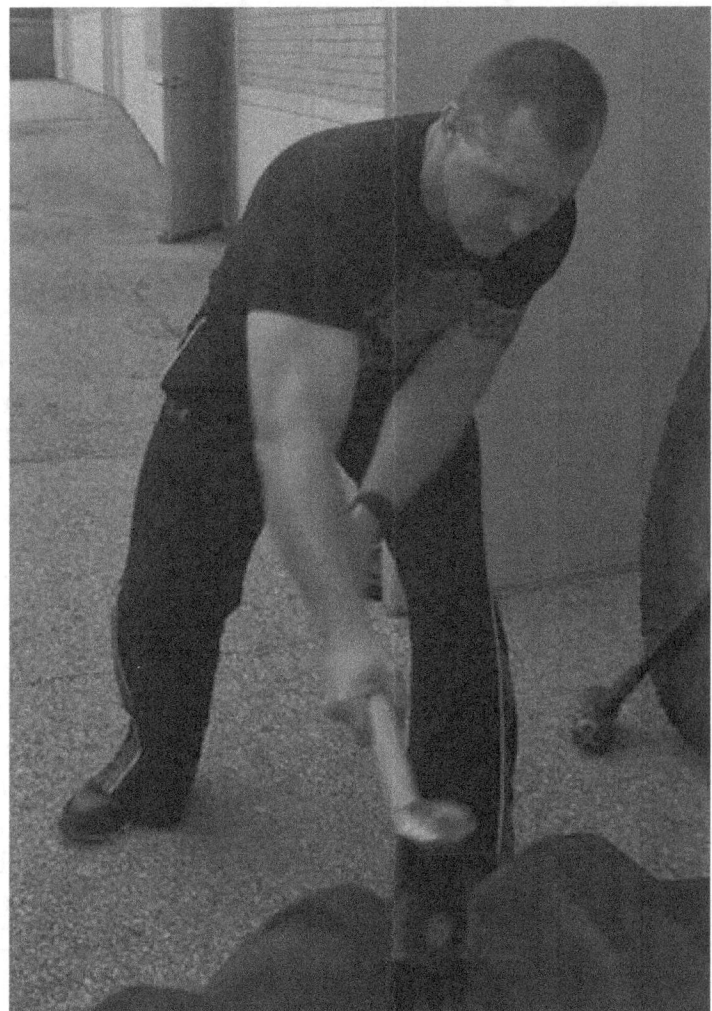

What made you a trainer?
Lisa Klaus-Ogden

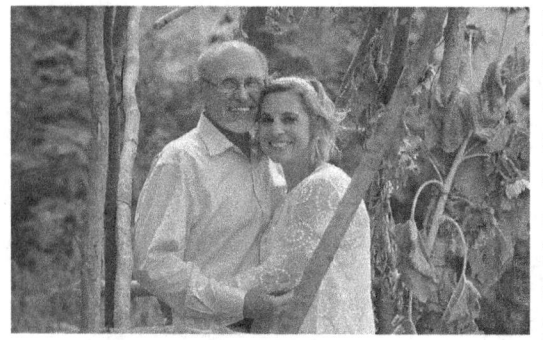

I started training 6 years ago after making a career change from agriculture. I have bachelors degrees in Animal Science and Agronomy, and a Masters Degree in Crop Sciences, all from the University of Illinois. I still live on the farm I grew up on in Illinois, where my family raises hogs, corn and soybeans. I am married to an amazingly kind soul, Eric. We have a beautiful 21 year old daughter that lives in Bloomington, IL where she lives out her passion of working with autistic children, and a fantastic 21 year old son who is in the Navy living in Spain. Could not be prouder of them!

I started training part time after spending about two years changing my life and losing one hundred pounds. I was overweight and unhealthy nearly all my life. I finally decided to do something about it when I realized I was not much younger than my father was when he had open heart surgery. I was on 4 prescription medicines for headaches and high triglycerides, and regularly took 12 Excedrin through the day. I had migraines at least once a month. I realized i was on the same path my father had been on leading up to his heart surgery, and it scared me. I slowly changed my food and started going to the gym early in the morning so no one would see me. Over time I realized I could actually do something about my body and my health. I started to do sprint triathlons, bike races and runs. I found I loved how my body felt, instead of hating how I looked. It took time but I lost the weight and found my passion along the way. I loved agriculture and helping farmers to be the best stewards of their land possible. However, helping others see their own potential, helping them to see that they are stronger then they think, that there's nothing they can't do, that they can live the best life possible and be the best possible version of themselves.....that is why I train. I wake up everyday excited to change people's lives. I work all day feeling high as a kite watching people work to be the best they can be. Seeing the little changes in people and their health....being able to better enjoy time with family, feeling capable, reducing medications, getting rid of headaches, having more energy to do things once not possible......it's what I get up for, spend time away

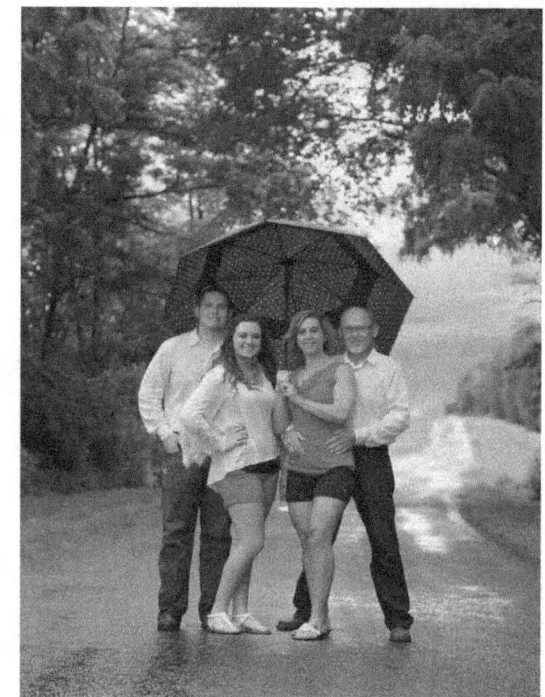

from home through the week for, work long hours for. It's what God created me to do. I am so amazingly blessed to do what I do everyday. I am blessed to work with the team I do and the clients I do. Most days I cannot believe this is my life.

What are your strengths? Weaknesses?

I believe my strength is my struggles. There is not much I haven't dealt with in my life. I have battled weight and health issues. I have fought food addiction, eating disorders, and depression. I have always struggled with food, even after I lost my weight. I sought out sugar like a drug addict. I have had to deal with an abusive relationship. I was a single mother with a full time job trying to get healthier. At one time I was a single mom, owned my own business, was working on my masters degree, led a 4-H group with my sister, was our county 4-H Federation leader, was on the school board and the County Foundation board, and made it to the gym daily. I get it! I am not walking in others shoes to know exactly how they are feeling, but I get the struggles.

What has your focus? What are your goals?

I try and focus on always learning ways to be a better trainer and finding new ways to challenge my clients. I want them to see and feel that they can do more than they think they can. I want them to learn to enjoy being active by finding things they enjoy doing.

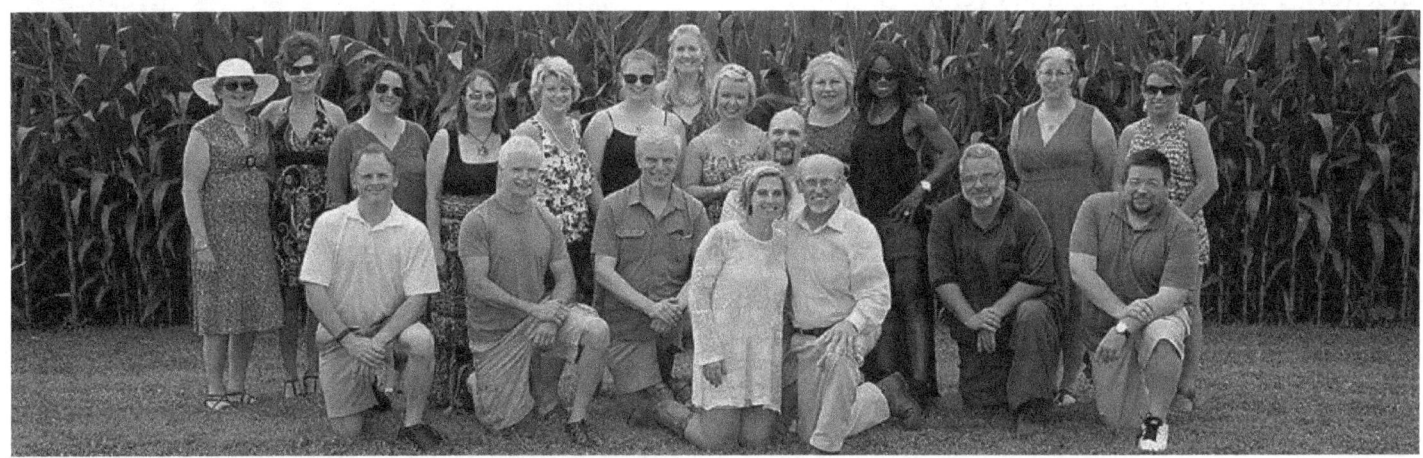

What is your philosophy on nutrition?

My nutrition is pretty strict because it has to be. Although I feel like it's been coming on for several years, in fall 2015 my immune system crashed. I have fought abusing food my entire life, and I feel that it finally caught up with me. Everything I ate my body attacked and made me sick, with terrible inflammation. I had lost 100 pounds and I had gotten to stage several times in bodybuilding competitions, but I don't feel that I was truly healthy. I still binged through those things. I was forced in fall of 2015 to really take my nutrition and relationship with food seriously. For several months my husband made me bone broth, kefir, turmeric tea, juice everyday. We took out anything that was potentially inflammatory. It took months and trial and error. I am still learning what my body does and does not like. I can get sick, extremely fatigued, terrible headaches if I eat the wrong things. I eat a lot less protein than I once did, vegetables, and healthy fats. I don't eat gluten, dairy, or sugar. My husband is an amazing cook and has discovered many seasonings and spice combinations that taste wonderful and don't cause a reaction. We don't go out to eat because there's always uncertainty what is being used in the preparation, and our food at home tastes so much better. We raise a lot of our own vegetables and chicken and I know where all my beef comes from. It's all been frustrating but a huge blessing as well. For the first time in my life I feel in control of my food.

Do you take supplements?

In addition to a strict food plan, I take vitamin c and vitamin d to keep my immune system healthy. I also take electrolyte tablets, magnesium, evening primrose oil, digestive enzymes and probiotic.

What is your workout schedule & why?

When I was going through my weight loss journey, i started to run and bike often. As I got interested in doing bodybuilding competitions, that evolved into more

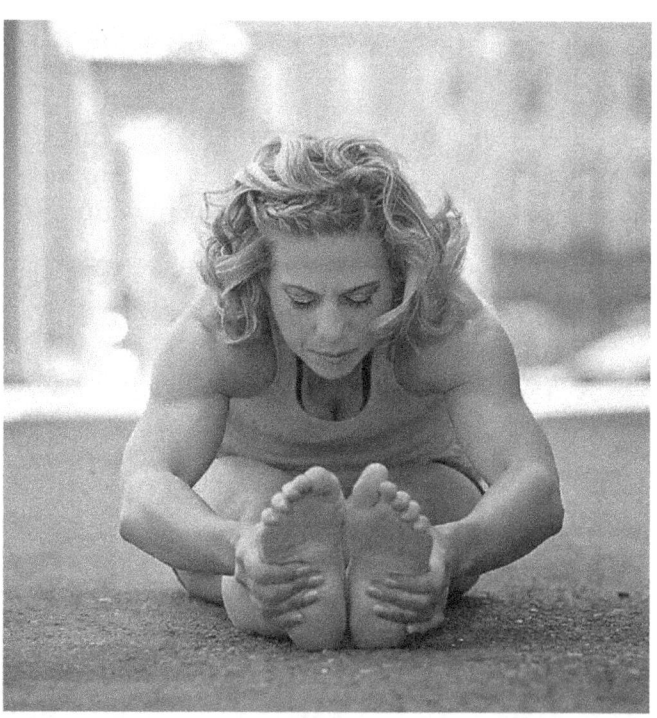

weight lifting and steady state cardio. Right now I try and get cardio in 5-6 days a week, through running or high intensity interval training. I do yoga at least twice a week, also try and lift 4-5 times a week. My schedule is busier than it used to be so I get what i can. Some days it's half hour of lifting and some days it's two hours. I just know mentally, spiritually, and physically I am best when I move. None of our bodies are meant to sit all day, but mind definitely isn't.

What does Train to Live mean to you?

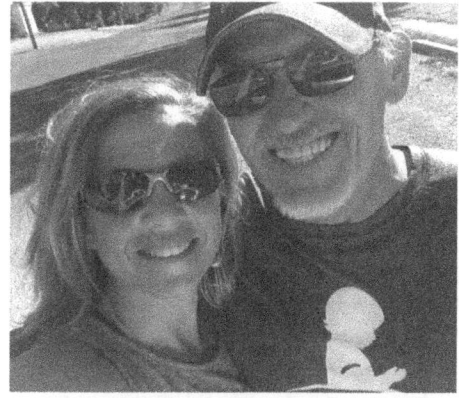

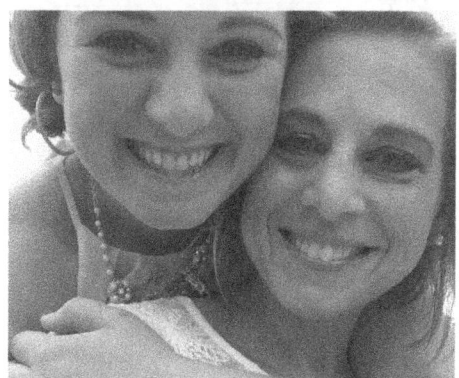

My focus has moved more to just enjoying the body God gave me and doing all I can to keep it healthy. Any free time I have I spend it with my husband running, hiking, biking, gardening, being active....taking advantage of what God gave us. My mindset has evolved from having goals to work toward to living the fullest life possible. I know how bad I can feel if I don't, and that motivates me everyday to keep moving. This is exactly what Train To Live means to me. Train everyday to live everyday. This isn't about short term goals, although sometimes those are necessary. This is about life. About feeling good. About being the best version of you. Everyday. This is a lifestyle. I believe Integrity is different because of that simple statement. Train to live. I get up everyday with the goal of teaching this and showing this to as many people as I can. This is my passion....it's what I think about when I get up and when I go to bed at night. It's what I don't mind losing sleep over, what I'd do if I didn't get paid. It's what I was created to do. I feel successful when someone gets it, when they realize they can do more than they thought they were capable of, when they understand food can either cure them or kill them, and they begin to make choices accordingly. Success is watching people transform mentally and spiritually as much as physically. I also feel successful when I watch my daughter live a full life with amazing priorities and when I collect bushels of vegetables from our gardens. I have attained success in my life because I have found my peace. My food and lifestyle choices have a huge impact on that peace. I absolutely believe everyone can attain that peace, and that Integrity can play an integral role in finding it. Integrity can help provide everything needed to refocus on yourself and your body's needs, everything needed to get your mind and body healthier than it's ever been.

Workouts that explain my style of training:

Workout 1
10 rounds
2 minutes sprint
100 jump rope
25 push-ups
Finish with incline treadmill

Workout 2
-Military press on smith machine *6 sets, 30 seconds rest between*

-Shoulder press, heavy weight as many as possible without rest......followed by a set of shoulder press at half the weight, twice the reps

10 reps each, 4 sets
-Leaning lateral raise
-Bent over rear delt
-Cable front raise
-Pike push-ups

Workout 3
10 reps each, 5 sets
Rolling skullcrushers
Bench dips with plate
Overhead extensions
50 rope slams

6 sets
V-bar cable Tricep pressdowns to failure, dropping weight on each set

10 reps each, 5 sets
Cable bicep curls
Db hammer curls
Preacher curls
50 ball slams

6 sets dumbbell bicep curls to failure, dropping weight each set

My favorite recipes:

Bone Broth
Approximately 6 lbs soup bones, cut 1"-2" thick
4-6 carrots
4-6 stalks celery
4 cloves garlic
2 tlb. Apple Cider vinegar
1 large onion

Brush bones with olive oil. Place on foil lined backing pan in single layer. Roast at 450 deg. for 30 minutes then turn over and roast an additional 30 minutes until bones are a deep brown. Place bones in crock pot with veggies. Put in enough water to cover bones by 1/2". Set crock pot on low and cook for 24 hours until broth is a golden brown. Remove meat, bones and veggies. Pour broth through a strainer into a large pot. This removes the food bits remaining. Place broth in fridge for 24 hours til fat sets up Skip solidified fat off and dispose of it. If the broth is congealed, simply warm until liquified then place in jars for storing. Broth will keep in fridge for 5-7 days!

Avocado Chicken Salad
2 - 3 boneless, skinless chicken breasts
2 avocados (peeled, pitted & mashed)
1 chopped celery stick
2 tblsp chopped cilantro1 lime
hot sauce

Cook chicken in crock pot, shred after cooking. Add mashed avocado, celery & cilantro. Squeeze lime juice and add zest. Top with your favorite hot sauce to taste.

Client Testimony:
-Dawn & Halle Douglass

I first heard about Integrity Training Systems and Debbie Portell while listening to a local radio station. I listened to her talk with extensive knowledge about their approach to personal training and overall health and I knew this was exactly what I had been looking for in a trainer. She explained how they have a trained staff that will evaluate each client for posture and muscle imbalances and that is where they start. They set up a workout plan specifically designed to correct those imbalances and build upon that. Due to some prob-

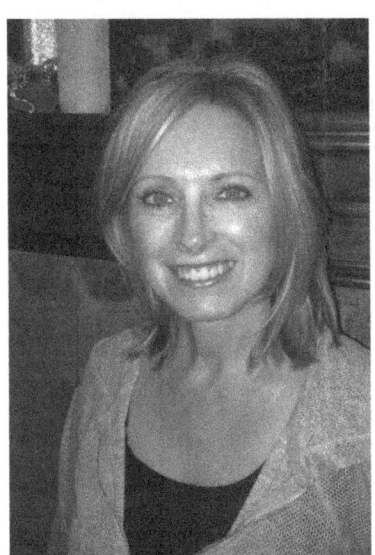

lems I have with my hips and back I had become inactive, which only made the problems worse, and I knew if I was going to try working out again, I had to work with someone who had the knowledge to help me. I asked my 15 year old daughter to join me and made the decision to call.

We made an appointment with trainer Lisa Klaus and our lives have changed for the better from day one! With our assessment, she was able to determine our individual weaknesses and form workouts to correct them through stretching and strengthening. Lisa empowers us each workout with her experience, her knowledge and her inspirational ways! My daughter, who wasn't really excited about coming at first, now looks forward to each workout as she gains confidence and strength. As for me, I have found a lot of relief from the pain I used to experience and have become inspired to take total control of my overall health by adding the Nutrition Program to my plan.

Integrity Training Systems is different than any other place I've tried. No matter what kind of shape you are in, you will come out a better you!

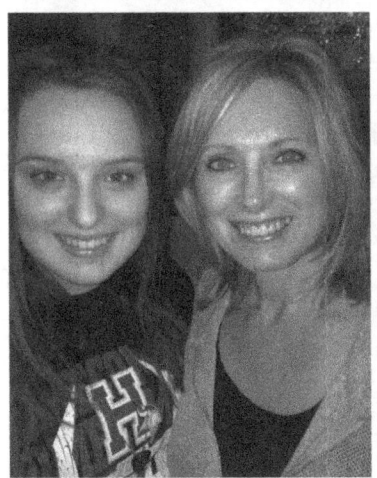

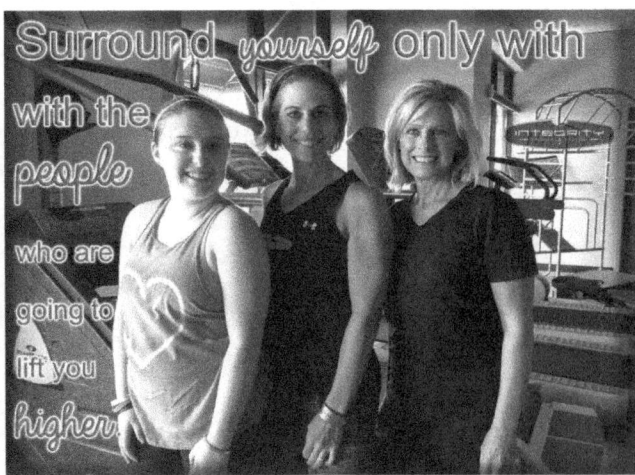

Client Testimony:
-Steve Gust

As a 52 year old with high blood pressure and three back surgeries, Integrity Training Systems has enabled me to "Train to Live" a better life. Integrity for me has meant a team with knowledge, understanding, passion, and inspiration. Lisa Klaus, my trainer, has enabled and empowered me to train properly utilizing the correct technique. She has helped me understand my physical weaknesses while motivating me to push past my limitations. Furthermore, she helped me identify my imbalances consistently modifying exercises to improve and strengthen my entire body. Most of all, Lisa listens attentively always asking questions to clarify and understand how I am feeling. Debbie Portell, my nutritionist, has taught me the proper foods to fuel my body for lifestyle not a diet. Her knowledge and understanding of how proper food selection plays a vital role in living a healthier life has enabled me to lower my blood pressure and live a life free of medications. I am living a healthier happier and more fulfilling life.

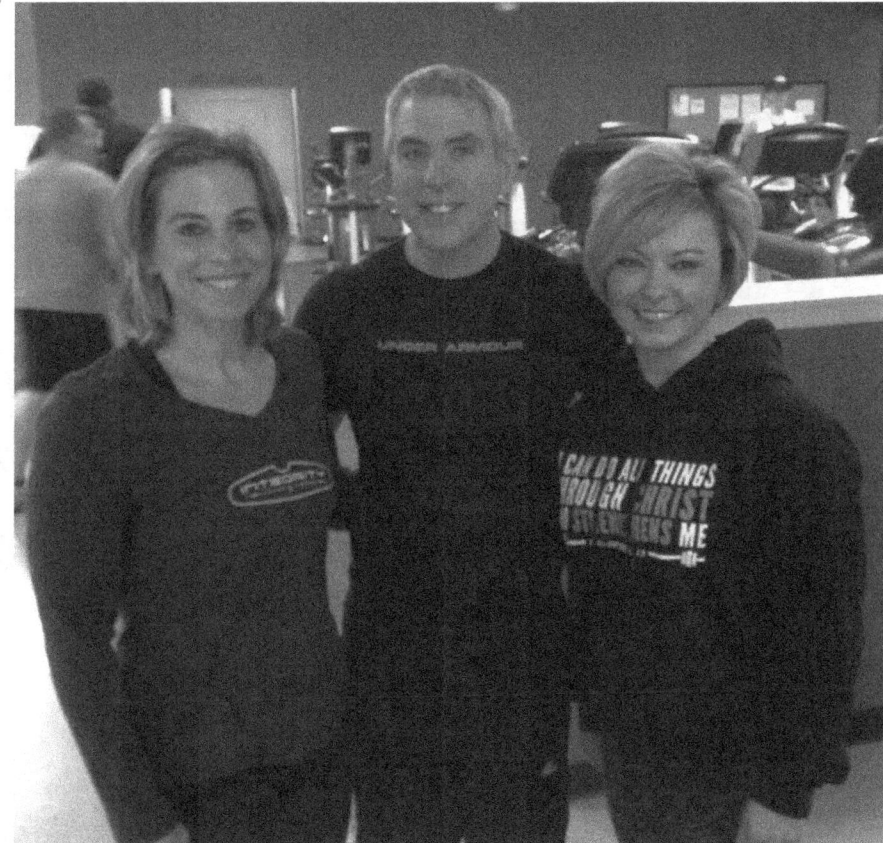

What made you a trainer?
Mike Harris

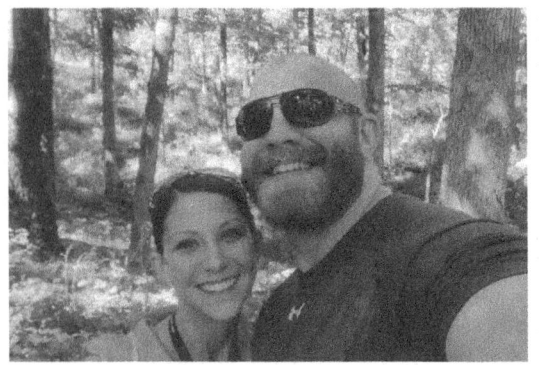

I have been an athlete for my entire life and have always enjoyed the training aspect of sports just as much as the competition of it, so that led to me developing a passion for the science of exercise and in particular, building muscle. I have always had an interest in advancing my own training and workouts, and that has led me to pursue a career where I can take what I know and learn, and then try to pass it on to others.

What inspires you?

Something that really motivates me to wake up each morning, (no matter how early for cardio) is knowing that whatever goal I am working towards, if I get up and put the work in I will get the results.

What are your strengths?

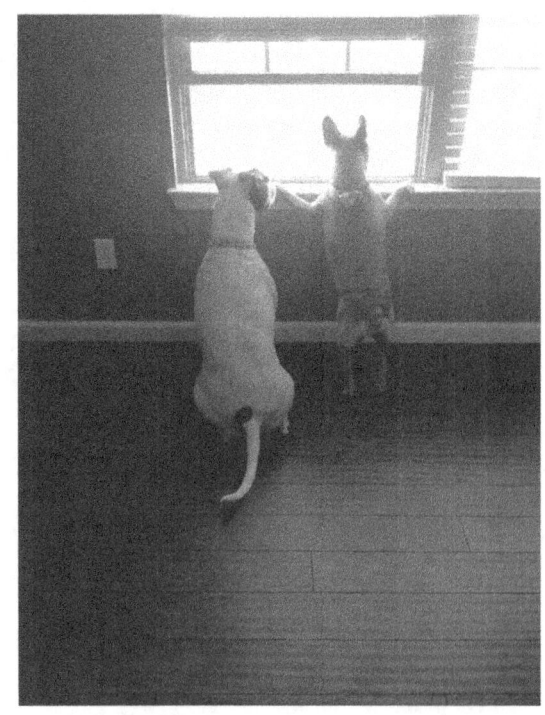

Attention to detail – I pay great attention to the little things about movements that make a world of difference in how you can feel and focus your muscles working and the small details add up to make a big difference in your development.

Passion for teaching – I very much enjoy being able to share my knowledge and love for health and fitness with my clients and really anyone who will listen. I believe the greatest tool anyone who wants to make a health and fitness lifestyle change can have, is information.

Weaknesses?

My main weakness is food. I grew up raised on fast food and boxed processed junk. I eat healthy to fuel my body towards my goals but I still struggle from time to time with saying no to crap.

Focus and goals:

I am currently preparing for my second bodybuilding competition having just recently won my first competition. My goal with competing in bodybuilding is to show my hard work, and the progression of my physique every time I step on stage. If I can improve every time, then I am successful.

What is your philosophy on nutrition?

Nutrition is the absolute most important thing in life, that the overwhelming majority of the population give no thought too every day. I could talk for days about nutrition but to keep it short and sweet, you can use food to do anything you want with your body and health.

My current Ketogenic Competition Diet
Meal 1
5 large brown cage free, grain free whole eggs

Meal 2
8oz 90% lean grass fed ground beef

Meal 3
6oz organic chicken breast
6oz avocado

Meal 4
6oz 90% lean grass fed ground beef
2oz avocado

Do you take supplements?

Supplements should be taken to "supplement" your healthy diet. I believe everyone should take a few supplements to ensure that your nutritional bases are covered regardless of your diet.

My supplement regiment:

General Health

Daily multivitamin (recommend for everyone)

Omega 3 fish oil (recommend for everyone)

Joint health supplement (recommend for everyone)

Vitamin D3 (recommend for everyone)

Sports Nutrition

Kre-alkalyn creatine (recommend for weight training males)

Branch Chain Amino Acids "BCAAs" (recommend for everyone weight training)

Glutamine (recommend for everyone weight training)

What is your workout schedule & why?

I have experimented with a lot of different styles and systems of workouts and I believe I have found what works best for me. My goal is always to grow muscle and I believe in lifting as heavy as possible with perfect form to do so.

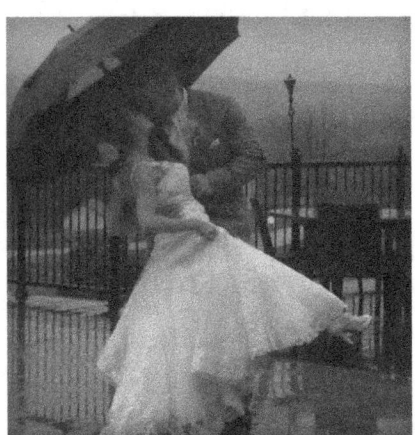

Monday: *Chest/Calves*
Tuesday: *Shoulders/Arms*
Wednesday: *Off*
Thursday: *Legs*
Friday: *Shoulders/arms*
Saturday: *Back*
Sunday: *Off*

What is your definition of passion? Heart? Success?

Passion to me is having a genuine love for something. It means that no matter what happens you never lose your fire for whatever it is you love.

Heart is one's ability to overcome, to work harder than would normally be thought possible. It takes a lot of heart to change your life and do something different than you are used to, but it is the most rewarding feeling when you will yourself to succeed. That's heart. Willing yourself to do what you thought was impossible.

Success for me is setting a goal that I at the time cannot achieve, and then in the process of working toward that goal, I grow and develop into the person who can achieve it.

How do you stay motivated to make this a lifestyle and not a goal?

I have dieted and exercised for a large part of my life, as well as I have been overweight and miserable for a portion of it. I can tell you from those experiences that if you want to be truly happy, it starts with making your health/fitness/nutrition a priority. I'm not talking about just when it is convenient or when you're motivated in January, but make it a priority every single day and you will be amazed at what happens.

What does Train to Live mean to you?

For me Train to Live stands for the idea that you have to think about, prepare, plan, put into action, and pay attention to your health and fitness everyday so that the other areas of your life can be as enjoyable and fruitful as possible. It truly is a lifestyle and not just a diet or limited time program.

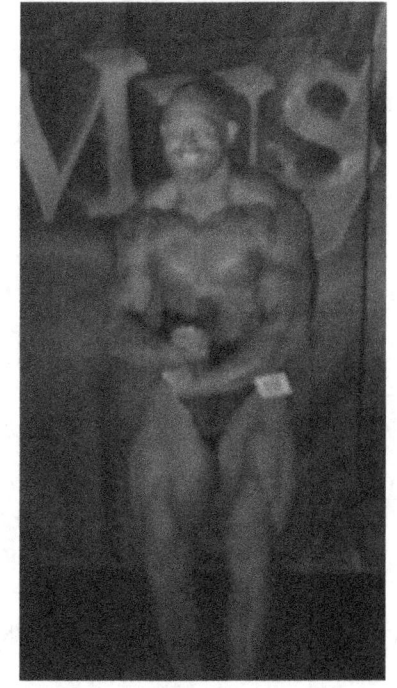

Client Testimony:
-Kimberly Simon

Breaking the Diet Roller Coaster

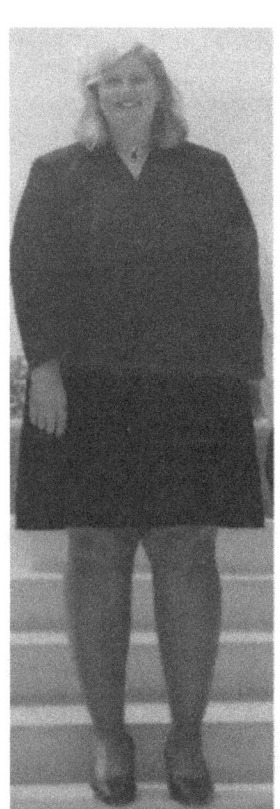

My weight struggles all began when I moved out of my parents' home after college. I thought I knew how to take care of myself, how to properly cook and how to be healthy…….boy was I wrong! My parents grew up with a farm to table mentality and always provided the best quality of food as I was growing up. But then I moved away and got a job and husband. Life got busy and we quickly learned the convenience of restaurants and carry-out. For a wedding present I received a bread machine and my husband and I tried every possible recipe, some of which included vegetables IN the bread --- that was healthy----right?   My weight slowly crept up, between being sedentary all day at work, watching TV at night, and finding daily restaurant "deals" every night of the week.   This one place had ½ price bagel burgers on Monday's………totally delish!!   Then I found out I was pregnant, what a delight AND an excuse to eat things I craved like breaded chicken and potatoes.   After my first child, I decided I needed to get serious and diet…..well one diet fail led to another.   After time, I was an expert at sticking to a diet for 6-8 weeks and losing 15-20 pounds each time and then gaining it all back and more.   This cycle kept repeating itself over and over again for almost 21 years.

Then I ran into someone at work that looked very "Fit", not skinny, but very toned and her skin almost glowed.   She looked healthy, she had definition in her arms, and she looked very happy. That was what I wanted.   She told me about Debbie Portell and her nutrition program.   I spent days researching and listening to Debbie's radio show podcasts.   I was sold and immediately called Debbie to sign up.   My family (especially my husband) was all like….there she goes again…another diet kick that will be short-lived, but somehow I knew this would be different.

My first 12 weeks was awesome! I felt better than I ever did and that 12 weeks led to another 12 weeks and then a year later I had lost 60 pounds and was feeling very proud and good with my accomplishments.   At this time I still had about 25-30 more to loose and it was getting mentally harder to keep the commitment especially when I was feeling good and was down to "normal" sizes in the store.   Then I started allowing a few "cheats" to reward myself. One cheat led to another and then I started gaining some of the weight I had lost. I still worked out consistently, but my mind was not dedicated to my food.

Then in January 2016 at 46 years old, I decided that enough was enough and I needed to first commit to my food and then secondly to exercise. I cut my exercise down and focused on my food 100%. Six months later I have dropped over 50 pounds and have reached my goal. Debbie and her trainers have been my support tools and I have surrounded myself with people that share the same values. I follow Debbie's nutrition plan, train in Integrity group training classes, and do Personal Training with Mike Harris, an Integrity trainer. For me, I needed the variety and to surround myself with people that would help me to succeed. Mike Harris with his no-nonsense and scientific approach was exactly what I needed. Not only did he ensure that my workouts were appropriate for me and my body type, but he literally got into my head mentally. Each session he would ask "how have you been?" and I always knew what he meant……"have you been eating on plan?". His caring, but no-excuse attitude really pushed me to do my best. I could literally hear his voice echo in my head on days I didn't even see him. I literally saw differences each week and he saw them too, which really kept it going for me. I remember the day when I was doing a push-up and actually saw my collarbone…..so exciting!!!! I was strutting around for days just watching it in the mirror.

The benefits have far exceeded my own journey to being healthy. I have set a family example for my husband and my 2 daughters. My husband went to the doctor for his annual check-up 2 years ago to find out that he would need to take statin drugs if he did not lower his cholesterol in 6 months. So he went to Debbie and after 5 weeks of following her program 100% his levels were normal. When he went back to the doctor the doctor said "I don't know what you are doing, but keep it up". He has been following Debbie's nutrition program and works out in her group training classes for about 8 hours a week. Then there are my 2 daughters. When they were both in high school they fell victim to eating sweets that was available to them at school. So when they started to gain weight, they asked if they too can goto Debbie. They both have lost over 30 pounds and know how the healthy way to eat as they goto college.

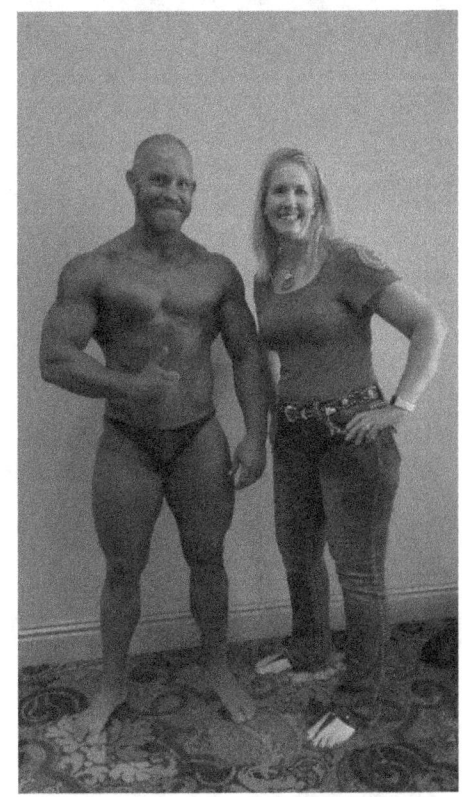

I am truly blessed to have Debbie, Mike and the entire Integrity Training Group in my family's life and mine. They have added not only years onto my family's life span, but we are healthy and can live life to its fullest.

Client Testimony:
-Mark Roberts

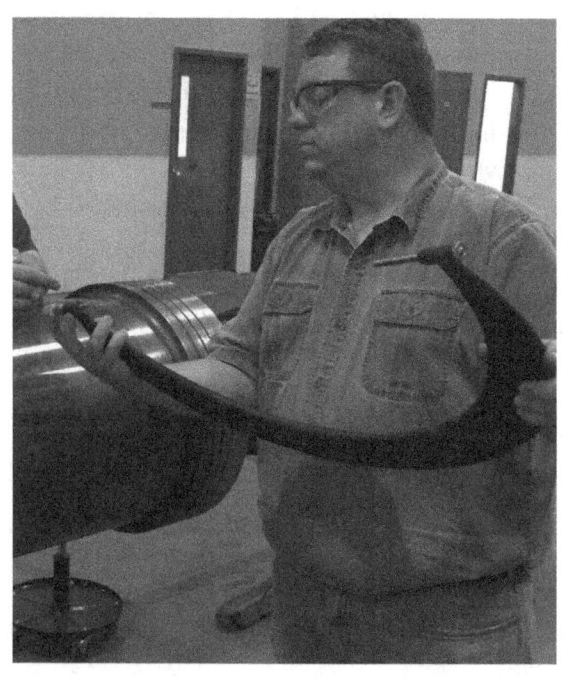

For the about the last 26 years, I have battled to lose weight and get in shape. I had occasional, short term successes that would ultimately end in failure and I would find myself heavier than I was before starting that particular effort. Over and over I would tell myself, "This is the one that is going to work", only to fail for any number of reasons.

As things were spiraling out of control over the years, my body would desperately hold on to a specific weight for a number of months and when it couldn't take the excess food and lack of exercise anymore, it would give and I would add another 10-15 pounds to what I was already carrying. This went on for years, along with occasional, half-hearted attempts to lose the weight on the next "diet" plan and magic pills from a local supplement store and even efforts from my doctor, prescribing pills to help curb appetite and promote weight loss.

The internal struggle I was dealing with had become a huge problem and no-one, not even those closest to me, had any clue how this was absolutely crushing me in my daily life. I became very good at hiding some terrible eating habits and dressing to hide what I was so ashamed of.

Then I stumbled across a radio show on 97.1 on a Sunday afternoon. When I heard the show, the things that were discussed always made sense to me. A lot of sense. I caught the show a few more times and wrote down the name and number they gave if you wanted to get more information about the things they were talking about.

I had that number written down for about a month before I finally called. Debbie Portell answered that call and spent about 30 minutes with me on the phone, asking questions about me that no doctor or other person that had attempted to help me lose weight had asked. Most of all, she was encouraging me, a person she had never met or talked to before, that we could solve this problem. I made that call in November of 2014. I did nothing with everything Debbie told me until June of 2015. I tried to get myself in the plan and for a variety of reasons (and probably some lame excuses), I finally made it to the Integrity Training Systems facility in October 2015.

After arranging everything with Debbie (and John Morris), I had an assessment appointment with Mike Harris, who was going to be my personal trainer. I had an appointment with Debbie the day after the assessment to discuss and implement a nutrition plan.

October 5th, 2015 is a day that changed my life. I met with Mike, a complete stranger at that time, to share some of the most difficult to discuss, deeply emotional things that only I knew I was battling. After a lengthy discussion about my struggles, my goals and the path to success we would tackle on the gym floor, we headed to the scale, something I had avoided for the last 6+ months because I knew the news would never be good.

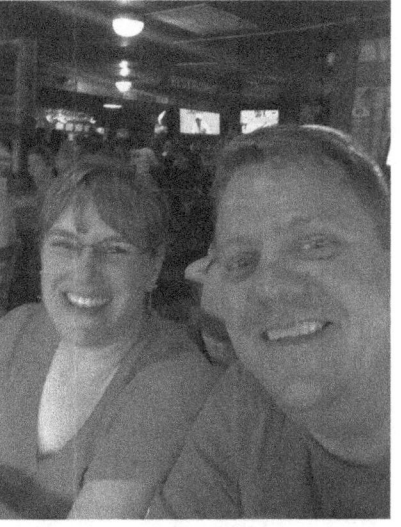

300.4 pounds.
I was embarrassed. I was ashamed of myself. I was humiliated that someone else saw that number. Mike looked me dead in the eyes and said "Don't worry about it, you're never going to see that number on the scale again". I'll never forget those words or the honest sincerity I felt he had in his intentions to make that happen.

I left that night feeling excited and a little intimidated by the physical work I thought I wouldn't be able to do. I was really looking forward to the meeting the next night with Debbie to see what the next steps were.

I brought my wife, Kristin, to the meeting with Debbie the next night, so I would have another person on my "team" that would listen, understand the nutrition plan and help me implement it. Just like the radio show, the plan made absolute sense to me and was very doable.

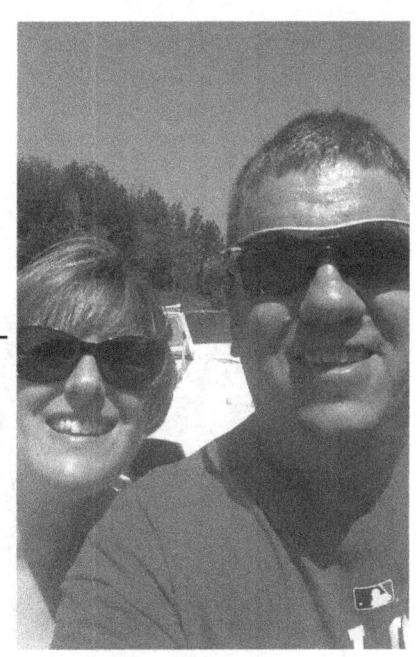

Once I got into this nutrition plan and working out with Mike twice a week, everything started coming together. I was feeling great. The weight was dropping off. Here's the thing though...I'd been here before, losing weight like this. Why would this be any different than all the other times I'd tried and failed? The answer wasn't simply Mike's dedication to teaching me the right way to lift or the most effective training plan to drop weight and get stronger. It wasn't simply Debbie's dedication to helping me make good decisions along the way as I was learning to make good choices while traveling or going out to eat. What made this work for me was the entire Integrity Training family. Everyone. From the trainers that weren't my trainers to the clients that I was putting in the work next to. Everyone in the building wants to see everyone succeed. The positive attitudes are contagious. The effects of a positive attitude are more powerful in my daily life than I ever knew.

So, here's the deal. On May 11, 2016 I stepped on the scale and weighed 197.4 pounds. On October 5, 2015, I set a goal with Mike, of losing 100 pounds. 7 months later, I accomplished a goal I never thought I could achieve. I have learned so much about myself, nutrition, weight training, goal setting and just stepping out in life and tackling something big, no matter how daunting the challenge is. Our capacity to do these things is in us. It just takes surrounding yourself with people that believe in you, pushing you, even when you can't see the path to success.

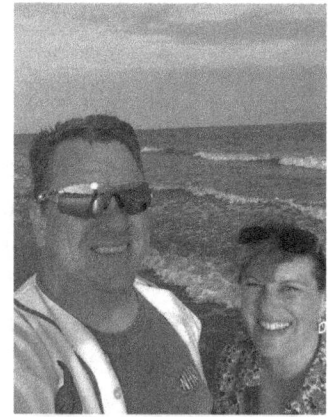

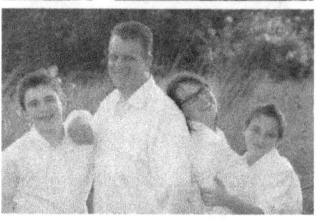

It's been 13 months since I started this journey. I am now down a total of 117 pounds and can't remember ever feeling better than I do now, both physically and mentally. I'm looking forward to seeing where I will be on October 5th, 2017 and what challenges I will tackle leading up to then.

I want to specifically thank my wife Kristin, Mike Harris and Debbie Portell for your dedication to helping me succeed. As I said above, it takes a family, but I really leaned on all three of you in the beginning as I started to make this life change happen.

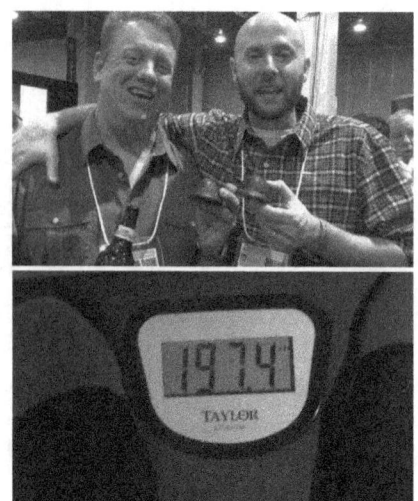
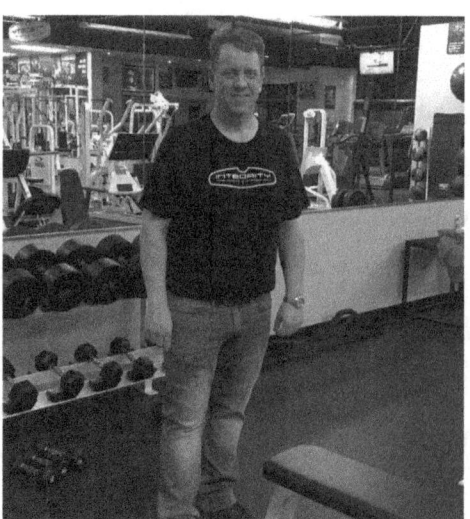
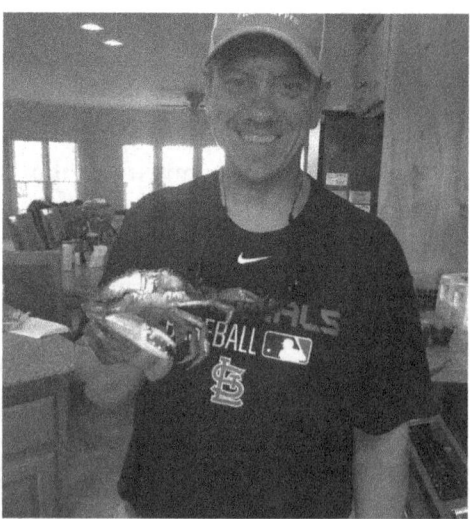

What made you a trainer?
Misti Weatherford

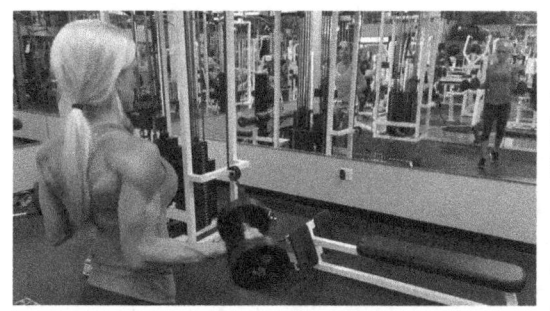

A few years ago I was working in the medical field, where I aspired to help others in every way I could. I worked as a dialysis technician, taking care of many people who were chronically ill.

The majority of my patients had high blood pressure and/or diabetes, which led their kidneys to fail. Most of these patients didn't realize what years of abuse to their bodies, in the form of poor diet and lack of exercise, was doing to them until it was too late. My patients would never again have functional kidneys and would forever be on dialysis. That is, until their bodies could no longer withstand it. The kidneys are such vital organs to a person's survival. And that's what my patients did on a daily basis – struggle to survive.

As a dialysis technician, my primary job was one I loved – to take care of people, while making them feel comfortable during the treatments they received on a weekly basis. I built amazing relationships with amazing people and heard so many stories from older generations of their decades of "living the good life," so it was always sad when someone's time had come and they passed on. During my many years in this job, I saw many people pass away. Again, it was just sad to me...and I always thought to myself, "I just wish there was something I could have done for them." This was when I first started to realize that my purpose in life was to not only help people, but to do it in a different way. Before they ended up like those I watched pass away. Before it was too late.

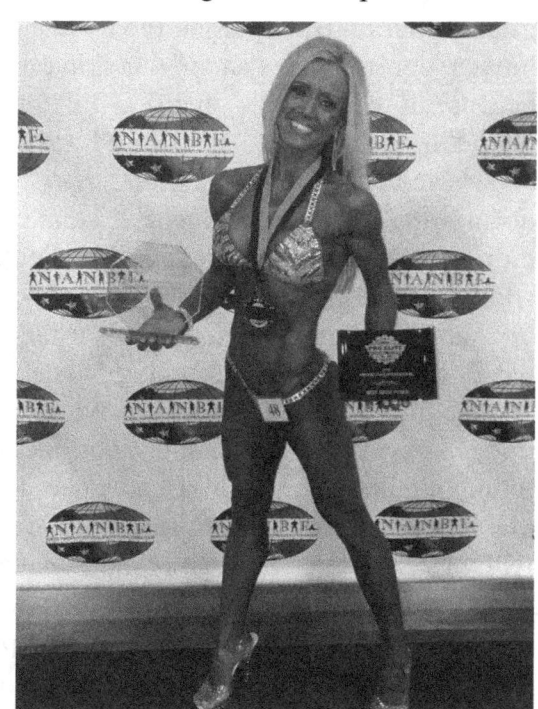

During this time, ironically, I had started to focus on some of my own personal fitness goals. I had always been an athlete in school and always in good health growing up. However, after having children and suddenly seeing my life's priorities change right before my eyes, I seemed to drift further and further away from the healthy athlete I once was. For me, I didn't like how I looked and felt and that made me realize I needed to change something. I needed to figure out a way to incorporate exercise and fitness into my life again. I knew that I didn't have to drift from it because of kids or being busy. I just had to do it. Especially as I worked a job every day where the effects of NOT doing it were right there in front of my eyes. I didn't want to live that lifestyle. I didn't want that to end up being me.

So, I decided to join a gym and hire a personal trainer to help guide me. And during the course of the six months that followed, I truly felt I had found my passion. I felt great. I felt strong. I felt empowered. I was taking control of my life again and transforming unlike I had ever imagined I could. I was doing more work in the gym than I ever thought I was capable of doing. I experienced breakthrough after breakthrough and, as each day passed, I realized more and more who I truly was, the person I wanted to be, and most importantly, what I wanted to do with it all. I had found my passion. I wanted to inspire and help people who were struggling to take control of THEIR lives again too, just like I did. It was then that I knew I finally found my purpose in life – to inspire and help people through fitness.

At this point, I knew I had to educate myself as much as I possibly could to help others reach their goals. I wanted to help others learn. I wanted to help others try. I wanted to help others find their own passion for life again. I wanted to just help others live! Because it wasn't just the physical changes I felt during my fitness journey, it was the mental changes as well. As I came to learn later, most people don't even realize the impact poor nutrition has on them. Our attitudes, our moods, our immune system, our skin...it's all effected because of the harmful, chemical-filled products people put in their bodies. The more I dove into training and started educating myself, the more I realized how devastating it all was, and worse – that people just didn't seem to know about any of it. People weren't educated on the negative impacts these chemicals had on them and how the body refuses to function properly when it's loaded with these things – leading to obesity and the great number of diseases we all hear about today. I knew I had to do something. And my heart was telling me that this was it. I knew people needed to know how important this information was and suddenly, I was excited about it all! And I wanted to be the one to tell them! THAT is the reason why I became a personal trainer – and that decision was probably the easiest decision I have ever made in my life.

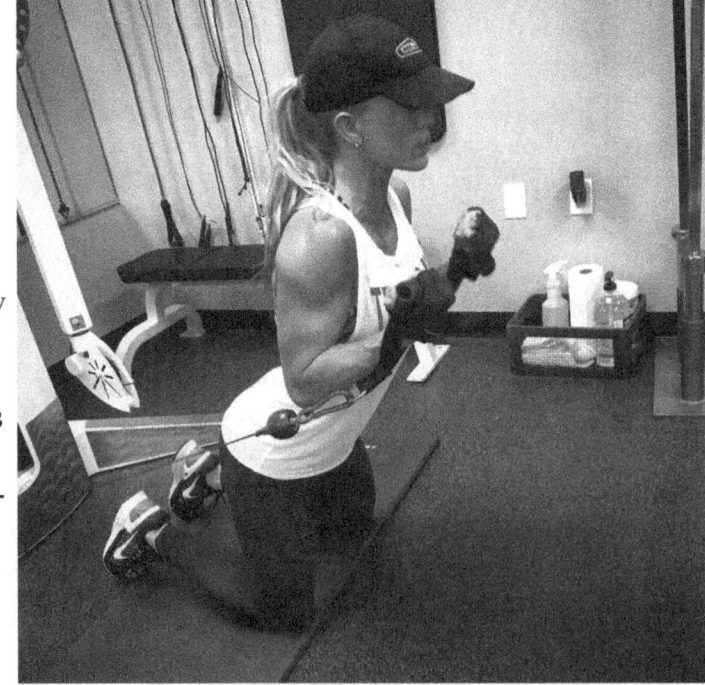

I have now been a full-time personal trainer for two years. I still wake up each day with a fire and a passion to walk out the door each day ready to help change someone's life. It's so exciting for me every day to drive to work and wonder who is going to crush what goal that day! Seeing the blood, sweat and tears pouring down and the look on people's faces when they crush goals and do things they never thought was possible is priceless to me. The most appealing thing about being a personal trainer is that there is no one formula that works for everyone. There is no "cookie cutter" diet or routine that works for everyone. My love for fitness rages because of the diversity in clients – from weight loss to injuries, to athletes, to those who have limited mobility, to bodybuilders – and every single day is a new experience that always brings a different level of excitement. There is no "one-size-fits-all" program. Working one-on-one with clients requires variation, preparation, specific technique based on personal factors, and constant evaluation. Even for the same person, there is always a time for adjustment and change. And in order to truly change someone with all this considered, it requires learning about them – learning who they are and what makes them tick. It requires learning about their goals, their mobility, their health history, their current lifestyle and their personal life. Everything plays a role in the desired outcome. In order to fully develop a program that's successful for each client, it must be customized for THEM, not just one plan you come up with for everyone. That's another thing I love about being a trainer. The job is what you make it – where creativity is key and every day is a new and different challenge filled with amazing and exciting opportunities for my clients...and for me.

The most rewarding part for me about being a personal trainer though, is establishing strong and lasting relationships with my clients. They all inspire me to wake up and become a better and healthier person myself every single day. I choose to live by our company motto, "TRAIN TO LIVE," every day. I choose to lead by example for my clients. To establish credibility. To earn their trust. They put their lives in my hands every day, and that's something I take very seriously. I pray every day that they find ultimate success on their journeys just like I did – but also pray that they find the little successes along the way too. That's what makes it fun. That's what motivates them. That's what makes them keep going. That's what changes their lives. That's what SAVES their lives. This is what I do. This is what I love. I can't imagine it being any other way anymore.

What are your strengths, weaknesses & goals?

My biggest strength as a personal trainer is that I truly live the lifestyle I preach to my clients everyday. I plan my meals and I exercise every day. I experience wins and losses just like my clients and also set goals for myself just like they do. I understand my clients. I know what they're going through because I live it too. So I can relate to them on those days when they "don't want to," or those days they text me saying they "really want those french fries." Why can I relate? Because some days "I don't want to" also. Because some days I "really want those french fries" too. I get it because I live it and when your client trusts you and knows you can truly relate to their struggle, a bond develops – and it's a bond of trust that makes them feel they can get through anything. It lets them know they aren't struggling alone. Exercising and eating a healthy diet is not easy. In fact, it's extremely difficult. But as we all say, if it were easy, everyone would be doing it. I listen, I sympathize, and I relate – but then I also reassure them that it will all be worth it one day...

...right before I make them start their workout. :)

I would have to say that a weakness of mine (other than french fries!) is that I still don't have a whole lot of years of experience behind me yet. I have such an extreme passion and desire to know everything there is to know about health and fitness and I try to learn something new every day. But there's still so much for me to learn – and there will always be something for me to learn. In this field, we are always growing and learning and I just want to be as fully equipped as possible each day to help change lives. So I live every day with my eyes and ears wide open to new thoughts, ideas and suggestions. The more I know, the more people I can help – and that's what I do all of this for.

What is your philosophy on nutrition?

For those who know me well, I have a saying that people often hear, and that is, "ok, my world can keep spinning now!" That usually is an indication that I have just eaten and my life can keep rolling on. I just need to eat to function, especially now that my body is running optimally and functioning as it should through a healthy and clean diet. Nutrition is my world, as I sometimes say to my clients. You just can't fuel your body properly and feel good without good nutrition. Everything inside me and around me is impacted by what I eat. Food can impact you physically, mentally, and emotionally. When I'm on a good nutritional plan, I feel like my body, my work, my family, and my whole world is wonderful. As soon as I get away from that, things start to suffer. The majority of people who don't make good nutrition a priority in their life simply can't recognize how it impacts their world on a daily basis. I truly believe that good nutrition adds life to your days and years to your life. For that reason, the first thing I say to a client who walks through those gym doors is that nutrition needs to be their number one priority. Because you can spend hours exercising in the gym, but without proper nutrition, you're just wasting your time.

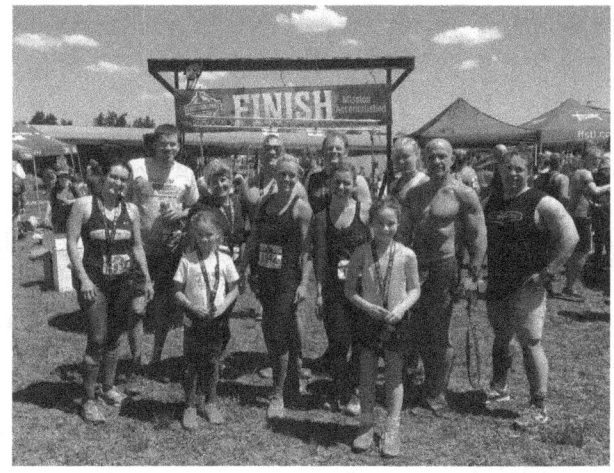

Everyone needs a good nutritional plan, but one that is tailored to them, their specific needs and their goals. Sometimes people have the misconception that if I eat what they're eating, I will look like them or feel like them. This just isn't true. Not everyone is the same. People often ask me about my own diet plan, but my goals are much different than most of their goals and I would never expect anyone to follow a plan that is designed for me. At the end of the day, I want each of my clients to be educated on a nutritional plan that can result in a consistent lifestyle for them, not a plan that is good until they reach a particular goal and that's it. The goal should always be to live a long and healthy life that is fueled by proper food and exercise.

Do you take supplements?

This is, by far, the number one question I get asked and I just love it. I am a professional bikini competitor and have done fourteen shows in the last three years. I've been very successful in my career and many have watched my journey. So naturally, everyone wants to know what supplements I take. And I get approached all the time by supplement companies about sponsorships. It's always so entertaining to see the faces of people when they ask that question, especially when I answer them with, "I have never taken any supplements and no I'm not interested! I have never taken supplements. I believe you can receive everything your body needs through good, clean, healthy food. To me, it's just extremely unnecessary and dangerous to put any chemicals in my body to help improve the way I look. My meal plan for competing is designed to give me all the essential vitamins and nutrients I need on a daily basis and it has been proven time and time again to be successful. It just takes hard work, dedication and consistency to reach goals. Supplements may give you short-term results, but create long-lasting damage to your body. That is something I don't believe in and would never be interested in for me or my clients.

What is your workout schedule & why?

I have been exercising 6 days a week (13 hours) for the past 4 years, rarely missing a workout. I am extremely consistent with my schedule and make sure I work specific muscle groups on specific days. I do this in order to reach the goals I have set for myself to be able to be competitive in the professional bodybuilding world. Some would say that the amount of hours I spend working out is a little insane, but it has helped me surpass the goals I set for myself both personally and professionally. It takes time, consistency and dedication to be able to be successful at what I do, and I will always give it all I have and set the example for those who watch me, are inspired by me and are trained by me. I don't expect my clients to do what I do, but if they have similar goals, I would definitely tell them what it takes. If their goals are different, the plan is developed to fit their goals. It's all situational and personal. My workout schedule isn't for everyone, nor would I ever expect it to be.

Here is my workout schedule: *(minimum of 2 hours/at least one hour per body part)*

Monday: *Arms/cardio/core*
Tuesday: *Legs*
Wednesday: *Back/shoulders/cardio*
Thursday: *Legs*
Friday: *Back/shoulders/cardio*
Saturday: *Arms/Legs/cardio*
Sunday: *Rest day (most important day, but hardest day for me)*

What is my definition of passion?

"If you can't figure out your purpose, figure out your passion. For your passion will lead you right into your purpose."

- *Bishop T.D. Jakes*

I struggled for so many years trying to figure out my purpose in life. I knew I enjoyed helping others, but struggled to find that one career that would truly allow me to give all I had to give to others. It all changed when I discovered health and fitness and its impact on my own life. I knew how it all made me feel...and I wanted that for everyone.

You see, passion is when you put more energy into something than what is required to actually do it. It's more than just excitement or enthusiasm. Passion is having the ambition, the desire and the mental fortitude to take action. Passion is discovering who you are and living out your purpose with as much heart, mind, and soul as is humanly possible. Passion is about discovering something that is bigger than you – and dedicating a life to making it better.

Fitness is my passion. Living a healthy lifestyle is my passion. Changing lives is my passion. I will always give everything I have to those who put their lives in my hands every day – no matter what it takes. This is what I do. This is what I love. What is your definition of heart?

This is always a hard one for me to define. I live my life by a set of values that is very important to me. That is, to work hard at everything I do and to always give my best. I've often been told that I put my heart into everything I do, to include my work. I don't do anything for recognition. I'm not driven or motivated by trophies or awards or medals. I'm just driven to always give 100%. I always have been. It just makes it so much easier to lay my head on my pillow every night knowing I gave everything I had and did all I could...no matter what it is. Give your all, do the right things for the right reasons and never give up on yourself, and you will be successful. If that's considered heart, then that's me.

What is your definition of success?

When I do anything in my life, I do it with all my heart and soul. I give everything I have. Not for the paycheck. Not for the recognition. And while the ultimate goal is always what you're shooting for, it's all the little things I experience and get out of the process itself that defines my success. Or the success of my clients. Whether it's me reaching a goal in my fitness journey, or a client reaching a small goal on their way to a bigger one, the process is full of successes – and those are the things I love experiencing the most. I love that I get to see such an amazing and diverse group of people – all with different goals – knock down walls standing in between them and their goals every day. It's truly a blessing for me to help each and every one of them find success, no matter how they choose to define it. To me, success isn't as much about crossing the finish line as it is breaking down those difficult walls on your way to get there. It's about the fight you have in you. It's about being resilient. It's about getting up when you've been knocked down. It's about continuing when things get tough. Sometimes, your biggest successes actually lie in breaking down those walls...before you even make it to the finish line.

How do you stay motivated to make this a lifestyle and not a goal?

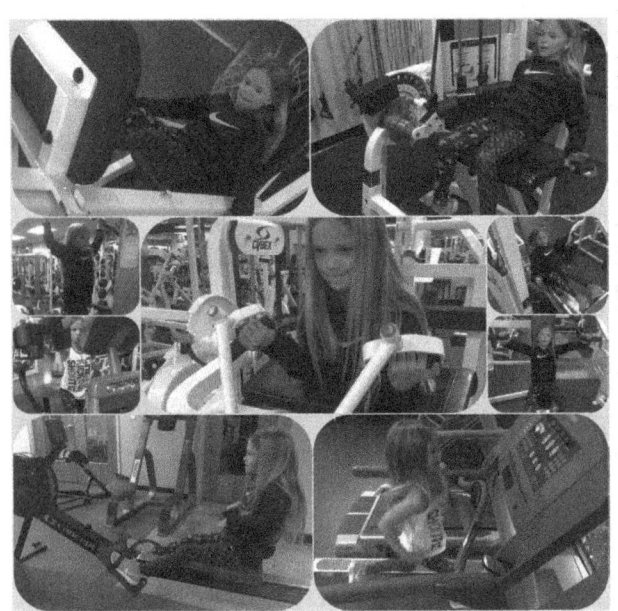

I want to lead by example every day. I'm motivated to show people that anything is possible – they just have to DO IT. I love being able to show people how to set goals and set realistic dates on when they can achieve them. Once we do that and they see that you really can accomplish anything you set your mind to, it motivates the. And that also motivates me! For me personally, I love being surrounded by amazing people who encourage me, push me and support me in my goals when it isn't easy. What we do is extremely difficult and adhering to a strict diet and workout regimen really takes hard work and true dedication. The motivation I get from my amazing support system is wonderful and I wouldn't be able to do any of this without them. In addition to that, I also read books and articles by inspirational people and listen to inspirational videos almost on a daily basis. These things also motivate me when I need that little "push," because the things they say and the way they say them are usually just what I need to hear at the time – and a reminder that I CAN do it and that anything is possible.

What does "Train to Live" mean to you?

"Train to Live" just embodies everything I've already said. It doesn't get much clearer than those three words. They truly represent what I do, what I teach and how I live. "Train to Live" is the motto in which I live my life every day. So, what does that really mean to me? It means waking up each day with a positive attitude. It means jumping out of bed ready to conquer the world and not letting anything stop me. It means waking up ready to do more, be better, and work out harder. It means being consistent. It means prioritizing my life in order to remain healthy for my kids and my future. It means eating healthy and continuously setting new goals to reach when the old ones have long been surpassed. It means never settling. I "train to live" to be the example for my kids, for my clients and for anyone who's watching. The impact that this motto has had on my life is so wonderful and I wouldn't trade it for anything. I want everyone to feel the same way. I want everyone to "train to live" as a lifestyle every day too...so one day, they can feel exactly as I do now too.

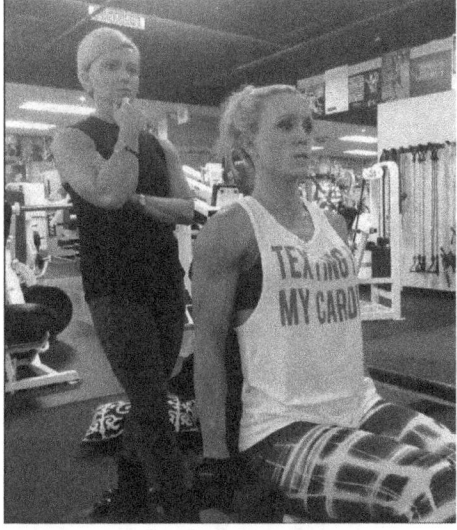

Workouts that explain my style of training:

Arms-*4 sets*
Standing EZ bar curls *10 reps narrow/10 reps wide*
DB hammer curls on incline bench *10 reps/ Standing for 10 reps*
Single arm DB preacher curl *10 reps each arm*
Band curls *20 reps*

Seated DB overhead tricep extensions *10 reps*
Flat bench skull crushers *10 reps*
Flat bench close grip DB press *20 reps* (go into press immediately following skull crushers)
Tricep push ups *20 reps*

Free Motion machine low bicep curls *10 reps*
Bench dips *20 reps* (elevate feet to increase difficulty)
Standing reverse grip DB curls *10 reps*
Dip stand dips *20 reps*

Bicep curl machine *10 reps*
Cable overhead extensions with rope attachment *10 reps*
Cable tricep press downs with rope 10 reps
1 min revers grip on Rower

Legs-*4 sets*
Leg Press toes over *20 reps*

Cable narrow stance squats *20 reps*
Sled Push 2 times down and back high/low push, high/pull back
1 minute sprint on treadmill

Single Leg press *20 reps per leg* (toes at top of pad)
Seated Hamstring curls *10 reps* w/2 count hold on bottom
Single Leg press down on assisted machine *10 reps per leg*
Forward walking lunges (carry DB's to increase difficulty)

Forward facing single leg Hack squat *10 reps per leg*
Leg Extensions *20 reps*
Wide DB squats *20 reps*
1 min reverse stepping on stairs

Back-*4 sets*
Cable wide lat pull down *10 reps*
Cable high row *10 reps* (use handles)
Cable wide handled seated row *10 reps*
Plank single arm DB rows *10 reps per arm*

Free motion machine reverse grip kneeling pull downs *10 reps*
Hammer strength machine reverse grip pull downs *10 reps*
Smith machine inverted pull ups reps
Pull over machine *10 reps*

Cable straight arm pull downs wide (use wide straight bar) *10 reps*
Back extensions w/ DB's. Perform DB high row when extending 10 reps
Wide pull ups 20 reps

Shoulders -*4 sets*
DB Arnold press *10 reps*
DB front raise
DB Iron Crosses
50 Rope slams
100 Jump rope

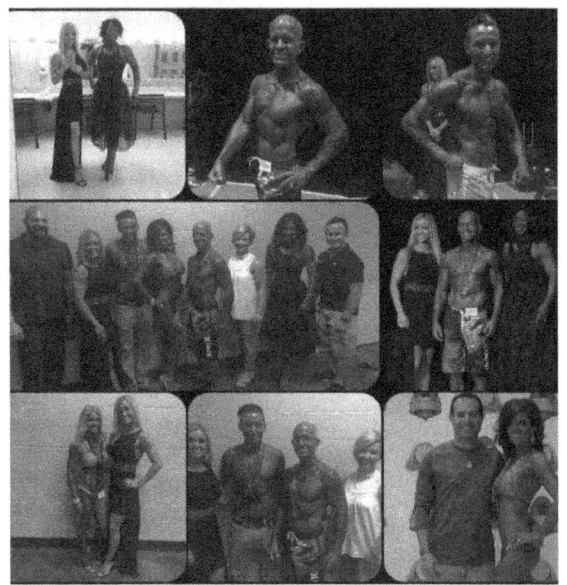

Barbell-military press *10 reps*
   -behind head press *10 reps*
   -upright row *10 reps*
Standing DB lateral raises *10 reps*
50 Rope circles (rotate arms counterclockwise)
30 Plank arm tap outs

Seated DB Knuckle out shoulder press *10 reps*
Seated lateral raises from side *10 reps*
   -followed by 10 partial lateral raises from side, thumbs out
100 Rope flutters

Chest-*4 sets*
Barbell incline bench press
10 reps, 8 reps, 6 reps, 4 reps
Smith machine decline press *10-8-6-4*
Incline DB press 10-8-6-4
Decline push ups *20 reps*

Flat bench DB close grip press *10 reps*
Flat bench DB flies *10 reps*
Pack deck machine *10 reps full 10 reps partial* out front

Incline cable fly *10 reps*
Chest press machine *20 reps*
Dip stand chest dips *20 reps*

Cardio
6 minute treadmill warm-up on incline of 15 (this is only performed once)
   -*2 mins* forward walking
   -*1 min* side stepping left
   -*1 min* side stepping right
   -*2 mins* reverse walling

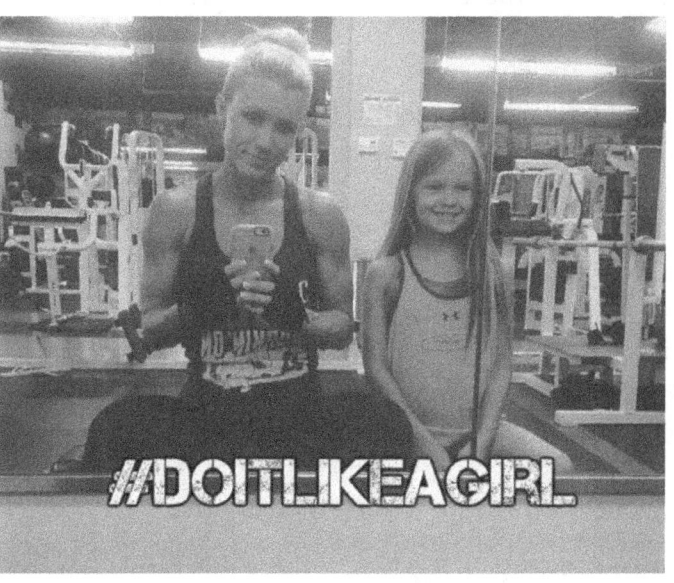

Make sure to lead into the following exercises on each line without rest. Once both exercises are complete, rest before moving on. After one complete round, do *100* jump ropes, before moving on to second round. Try for *3 rounds*.

50 Rope slams--->into 1 min plank hold
20 alternating step -ups on box or bench----> into 20 crunches
20 push-ups---> into 20 sand ball slams
20 air squats---> into10 jumping squats
20 jumping jacks--->into 20 lying leg lifts

My favorite quotes:

"Success is a journey, not a destination. The doing is often more important than the outcome."
-*Arthur Ashe*

"It is a shame for a woman to grow old without ever seeing the beauty of which her body is capable."
-*Socrates*

"Make your life a masterpiece; imagine no limitations on what you can be, have or do."
-*Brian Tracy*

"I survived because the fire inside me burned brighter than the fire around me."
-*Joshua Graham*

"Instead of giving myself reasons why I can't, I give myself reasons why I can."
-*Anonymous*

"A flower does not think of competing to the flower next to it. It just blooms."
-*Zen Shin*

"Set your life on fire. Seek those who fan your flames."
-*Rumi*

"You were put on this earth to achieve your greatest self, to live out your purpose, and to do it courageously."
                                                                -Dr. Steve Maraboli

"Destiny is not for the comfort seekers. Destiny is for the daring and determined who are willing to endure some discomfort, delay gratification, and go where destiny leads."
                                                                -T. D. Jakes

"You were born a winner, but to be a winner, you must plan to win, prepare to win, and expect to win."
                                                                -Zig Ziglar

Why should you choose Integrity?

Integrity Training is an example for all fitness businesses to follow. In fact, it's hard to even call it a "business," as we are all family. We work hard together, we laugh together, we cry together, we lean on each other, and we trust each other. We've experienced successes and failures together. We've all done things we never thought we could do. We've surprised ourselves...and others. But when all is said and done, Integrity is about YOU. When you become part of our family, your life becomes OUR life. Your dreams become OUR dreams. Your goals become OUR goals. We have a vested interest in every single person who walks through our doors and chooses to be a part of our family. We are Integrity...and we stand firm every day on what we teach, what we believe and what we live.

Train to live. You won't regret it.

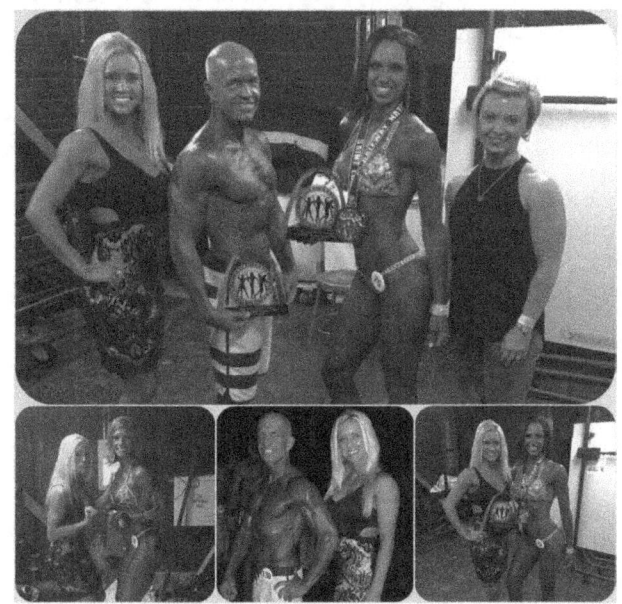

Client Testimony:
-Dr. Greg Luerding

The toughest part of training is getting started. So many people find themselves wishing they had started working out or eating healthy 6 months ago. Start now. Everyone starts this journey as a beginner. Without someone knowledgeable and experienced by your side, a coach, trainer, mentor or advisor, whether you're a novice or professional, you will never reap the maximum benefit from your efforts. This is where Misti Weatherford and Integrity Training Systems excels.

For 30 years I've been an avid runner. During this time my personal fitness goal was to become as healthy as I could by running and eating right. I found myself feeling weaker. Joining a gym didn't help much so I decided to work with a trainer, Misti Weatherford. With Misti as my trainer and Debbie Portell as my nutritionist I have become healthier than I've ever been. These 2 are world class. Having reached a level of fitness I never thought I'd achieve, I feel healthier and stronger than ever.

If you're interested in being stronger, healthier or more fit than you are now, contact Misti Weatherford with Integrity Training Systems. As a client, I work with Misti and have seen her change people's lives and transform their bodies. Seeing people start training with Misti and eating healthy lose over 100 pounds is not unusual at Integrity Training Systems. Other clients have gone from average Joes to looking like their bodies have been photo shopped. It doesn't matter if you're sedentary and overweight or a professional body builder. No matter what your degree of fitness or experience, Misti Weatherford with Integrity Training Systems can move you to the next level.

My advice to anyone looking to improve their physical appearance, health and or conditioning: contact Misti Weatherford. Take the first step.

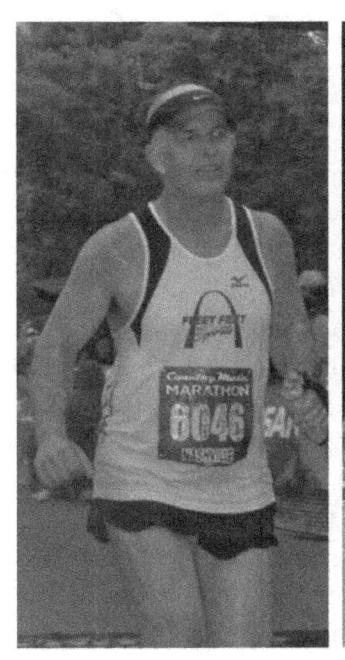
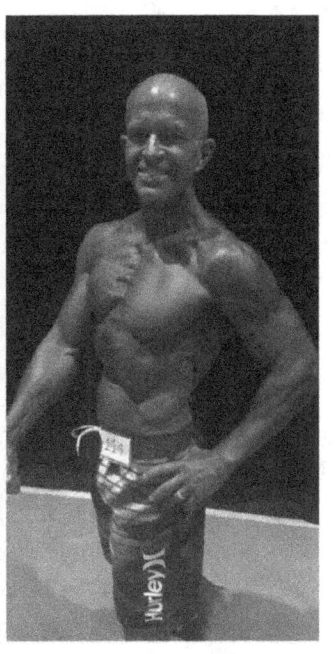
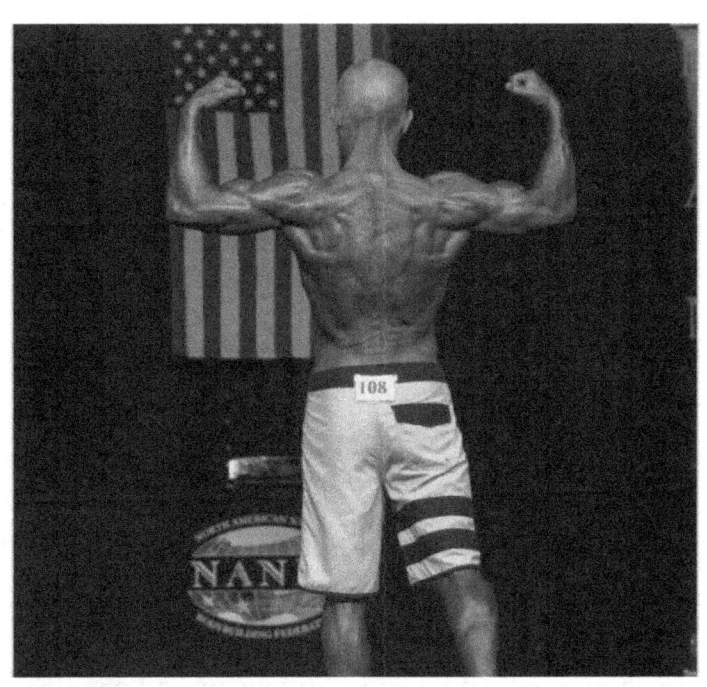
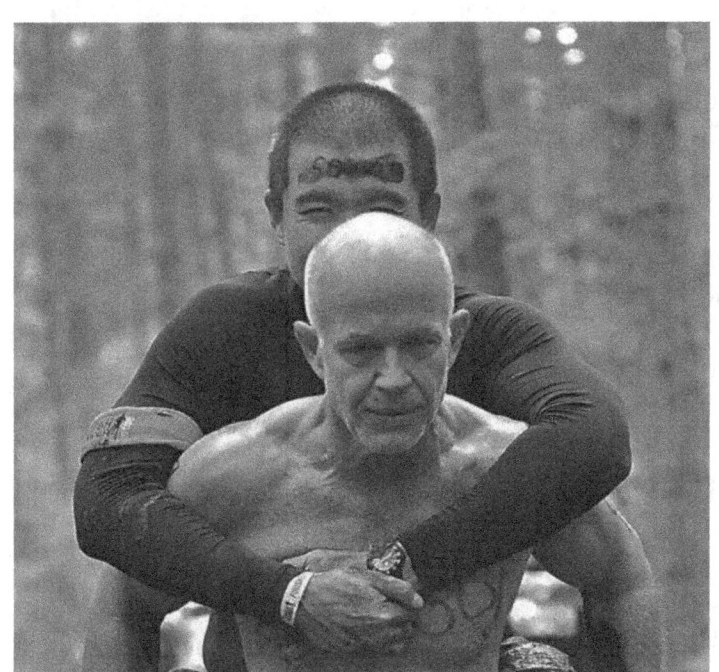
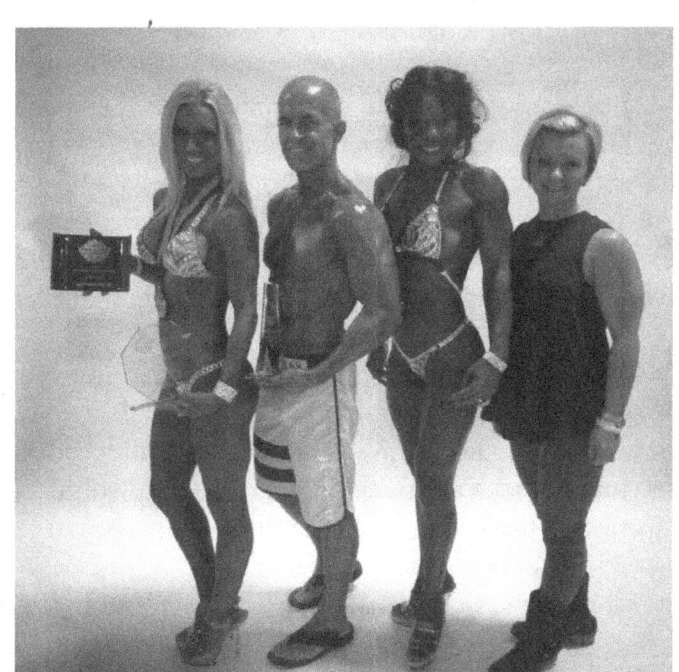

What made you a trainer?
Forrest Boston

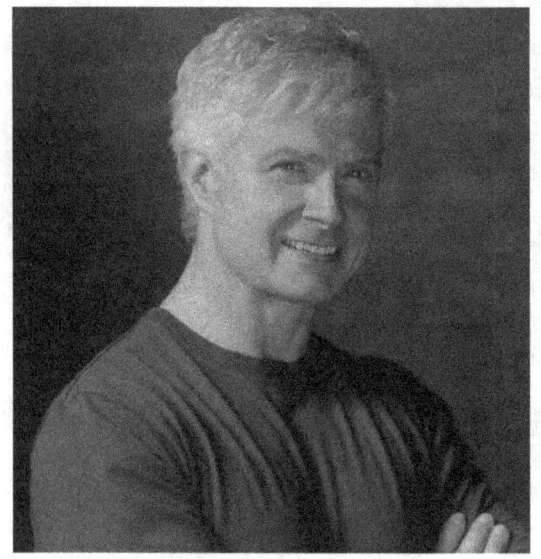

"I'm never going to be fat!" I announced to my parents. I was ten years old. Sometime after that, I finished my dinner and had a huge bowl of ice cream...with lots of chocolate syrup on top. As soon as I took that last bite, I began to feel guilty. I ran outside, pulled up my shirt, and looked at my reflection in the driver's side door window of my dad's car. I watched my belly as if it was going to do something besides go in and out as I breathed. It didn't, but I was examining it like a detective looking for clues. Was I already fat? I suppose I convinced myself I was, or at least getting there. So, I did the next logical thing. Around the perimeter of our 2.5 acre yard, I put up obstacles; a wheel barrow, a lawn chair, a push lawn mower, anything that I would have to either run around or climb on. I even used permanent structures like our two tool sheds. I commenced my routine, climbing up and jumping off the roofs of the two sheds and running around the perimeter going over all the obstacles I had strewn about. I did this for at least a half hour, maybe more.

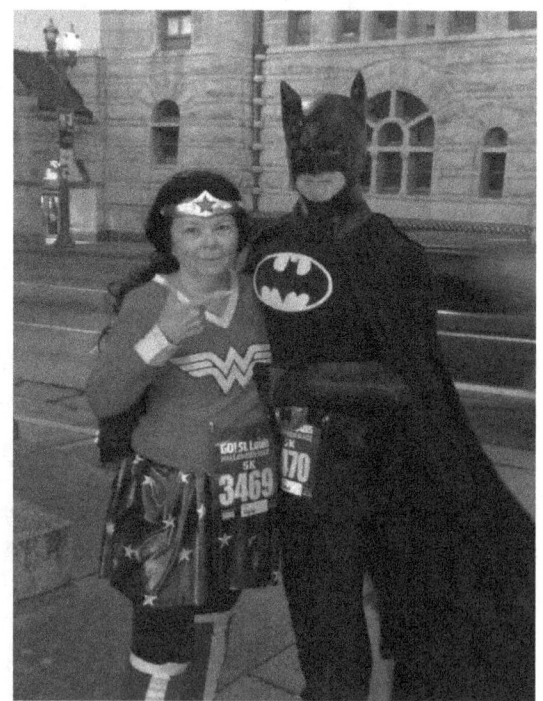

I suppose a lot of people would look upon this behavior as rather OCD. Could be. On the other hand, perhaps I was destined to be a trainer. I think all trainers, and other people who want to perfect a craft, whether it be health and fitness, music, a work of art, whatever, tend to lean towards the OCD end of the scale because we want our craft to be as perfect as we can humanly make it.

My dad wanted me to get into strength training years before I did. He did succeed into getting me into martial arts. After practicing in taekwon-do and hapkido for a couple of decades, it dawned on me that perhaps my punching and kicking would be better if I was stronger. That's when the strength training began.

It did improve my skill and performance and I also liked the way I was feeling...and looking. I began to get compliments in the gym and at work on how I looked. I have to admit, that felt really good and all of this was like throwing gasoline on a fire. Up to this point, all of my weight lifting knowledge came from books and knowledge I received from asking other people in the gym. The thought occurred to me, "I wonder if I could make a living at this?" That's what started my journey to becoming a personal trainer. And I have to admit, part of it was selfish. I wanted to improve my knowledge on how I could workout better and improve myself more. But that quickly changed.

I used to teach school for a living and I lived for that "Aha!" moment that you see in a student's eyes when he or she finally gets a concept you are trying to get across. I still live for that moment. When one of my clients gets the right form doing a squat or a bench press or some other exercise, that's exciting. Even more exciting is when they tell you how their lives are changing for the better: "I feel stronger." "That little bulge around my middle is going down." "People at work are telling me how great I look."

These kinds of things make me feel good, but then I get these other little nuggets from time to time that tell me, with God's help, I'm really making a difference in people's lives. My clients tell me: "I wasn't able to do that before and now I can." It may be getting up from the floor without assistance, or pain, or just being able to put a heavy box on the top shelf of their closet. The one I will always remember was an elderly gentleman who was having trouble with his balance and was afraid to walk down the hard, tiled corridor of his office building fearing he would fall and injure himself. He made my day when he came into this one particular training session and announced, "Today, I actually felt like skipping down the hall." Skipping!

I suppose what gets me up and keeps me passionate about this job, no, career, no service, is that - helping people and the joy I receive from it. So, I suppose it's still a little bit selfish, but not totally. After all, it is a win-win situation.

What are your strengths?

When a person asks me what my strengths are, I immediately become a third grader fumbling around in front of a classroom – stumbling on my words, looking at the floor, searching for something, ANYTHING, to say. I'm really a shy guy and I was always taught to be humble so telling my strengths feels like bragging. But, here goes.

I feel I'm very disciplined. If I want something, I'll study how to get it and then I jump in with both feet to do the work to accomplish it. Which leads me to strength number 2...

I'm very tenacious. I will not give up until I've achieved those goals.

I'm compassionate, sympathetic and empathetic. I listen to people, to their problems and want to help them. I care for people and strive not to judge anyone. I suppose that's why I took graduate work in counseling and was a counselor for some time. This is a good segue to my weaknesses.

Even though I strive very hard to be empathetic and understanding, and I work really hard to achieve my goals, I have to keep pride in check. Pride leads to another weakness, impatience. I have to keep telling myself that people come from different walks of life and different situations. I don't know everything about a person I see at face value. I have learned, if I can, to talk with a person and get to know them and what their story is. If I know them and understand where they are coming from, then I can be empathetic and understand why they are a certain way. This really comes in handy when dealing with clients – getting beneath the surface and seeing what makes them tick so that I can better help them.

All this, in a weird sort of way, leads to what my goals are. Of course, I want to be the best I can be physically, mentally, socially, emotionally and spiritually. And, I want to help my fellow human beings to achieve their goals also. This drives me to be the best trainer I can be, the best husband I can be, the best father I can be and the best person I can be. Ultimately, and in the proverbial nutshell is this: I want to help people to have the richest, most abundant lives they can have. Physical fitness and training is part of that. Education and empathy are the vehicles for that. And that takes many forms: one on one talking with people, working side by side with people in whatever situation they are in, writing, speaking, video, movies, blogging, social media. Going to people wherever they are at in whatever situation they are in and helping them. I still enjoy seeing that "Aha" moment.

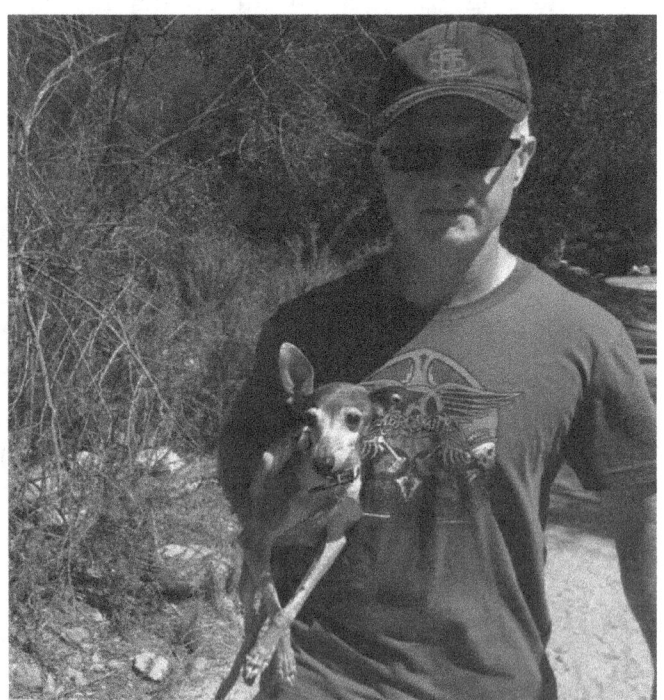

What is your philosophy on nutrition?

I am a science nerd. I love science. True, read: empirical, science is gaining knowledge, that is, facts, by observation. Hence, when it comes to nutrition, as in physiology, anatomy, psychology, kinesiology, and all the other -ologies that comprise our scope of understanding our human being, we need to gather facts and then use wis-

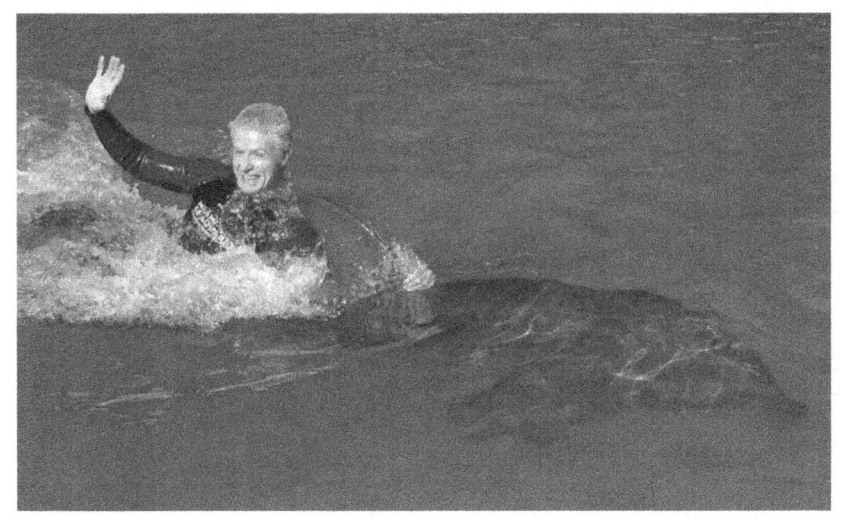

dom to apply those facts in order to obtain and maintain the best life possible.

I believe Hippocrates said it best. You know Hippocrates, he's the guy that has that oath that medical students take when they become doctors. He was a physician himself back in ancient Greece. In fact, he is considered the "Father of Western Medicine". Yeah, that guy said, "Let food be your medicine." How many of you have had your doctor tell you ***that*** when you went in to see him or her? Probably not many, if any at all. But he had it right. If you eat right, that is, whatever you put into your body, providing it's healthy and beneficial, will help you physically and mentally. It will heal you and keep you healthy.

When I began my journey to be in the best physical shape I could be in, and subsequent to that, when I became a personal trainer, I searched for how I could get this information on nutrition into my own brain as well as into the brains of my clients. The problem is, it can be quite involved and complicated.

I came across Bill Phillips' book, *Body for Life*. This was my fitness guidebook when I first started my physical training. Some of the concepts I still adhere to but what I found most valuable in it was his eating plan. It's simple and fairly easy to follow. I still use it as a backbone to my nutrition, although, I've modified it somewhat now that I have further education in this matter. But basically it's this:

Eat 5 or 6 meals a day. Each meal contains a protein and a carbohydrate. Eat vegetables with at least two of the meals. A serving is the size of your fist. Now, like I said, I've modified this to fit my goals tweaking it here and there as needed and I do the same for my clients.

Two points I strive to make with my clients are 1) 70 – 80% of the battle of the bulge is how you eat because a person cannot outwork what he or she eats and 2) Healthy eating doesn't have to be boring, tasteless eating. Here are a couple of recipes that are my favorite meals. They are, and I apologize for sounding like a commercial here, good and so good for you:

My favorite recipes:

Rice & Beans:
     Don't let the simple titles of these meals fool you. They are delicious! Also, it is suggested to use an iron skillet when preparing both of these dishes for better flavor.

1 Whole onion, chopped
1 Turkey Polish sausage, cut into small pieces
2 Cups brown rice, wild
1 Can black beans
Hot sauce (optional)
Cooked, chopped broccoli or mixed vegetables, fresh or frozen

Saute onions with turkey. Add rice and black beans. Cook over medium heat approximately 10 minutes. Add vegetables and let simmer for about 5 minutes.

Chicken & Brussels Sprouts
    2 or 3 Chicken breasts cut into bite sized pieces
    1 Whole onion, chopped
    Fresh Brussels sprouts, chopped and salted
    McCormick Garlic and Herb seasoning

Saute chicken and onion adding salt and seasoning. While this cooks, chop Brussels sprouts and add to chicken. Cook until sprouts are tender and chicken is done.

Do you take supplements?

Before we jump on the GNC bandwagon, go back and read the quote from Hippocrates I mentioned in paragraph two of the above section. Never mind, I'll save you the trouble and write it here as well – it bears repeating, "Let food be your medicine." First and foremost! Burn this into your brain! You can take all the protein and creatine and gobble down the hot pill or drink that is all the buzz on the internet or your favorite supplement store but if you are not eating the right quality and quantity of real food, those supplements aren't going to do you a lot of good. Look at the word "supplement" itself. They are items you are supposed to use to *supplement* your real food meals.

Now I'll step down off of my soap box. Having said all of that, the foods we eat today are not as nutritious as foods people ate back in the 30s, 40s and 50s. Industrial farms have come in and planted cash crops that have depleted the soil of minerals and nutrients that were in it at one time (OK, you got me. I still have one foot on my soap box). Therefore, it is necessary to supplement our food to get complete nutrition.

To begin with, get your meat, eggs, vegetables, etc. from private farms if you can. Eat grass fed beef, eat chicken and their eggs which are free range, eat vegetables not sprayed with harmful chemicals, and etc. Beyond that, I take a multi-vitamin to make up, or supplement, the food I eat.

I also take fish oil because, being a westerner, fish is not a major part of our diet. I try, but I don't always eat the amount of fish I'm recommended to eat (at least two meals a week). And Omega 3 is an essential fatty acid we get from fish that is vital to our health.

That is about it as far as my supplements are concerned. I do drink a protein shake as a recovery "meal" after my workout because I am wanting to build muscle. I have tried creatine in the past but I know that there is a certain section of the population that is immune to its effects and I think I fall in that category. But, I still try it from time to time.

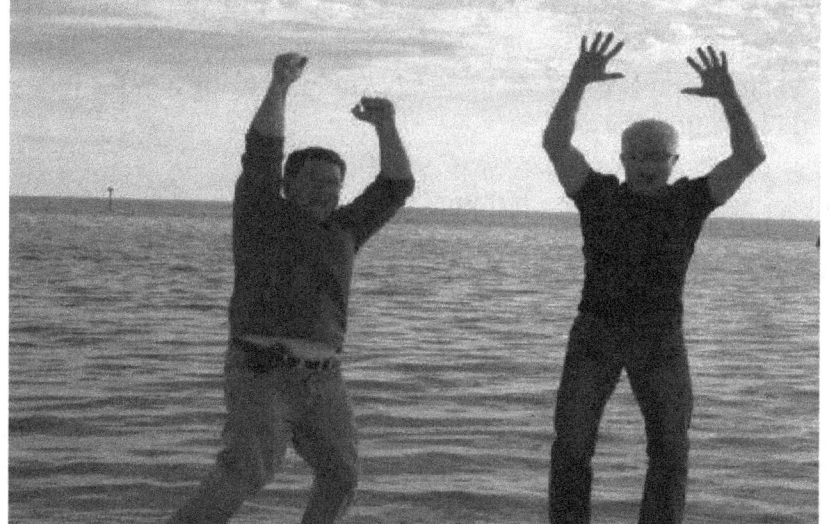

What is your workout schedule & why?

As I stated above, my base workout came from Bill Phillips' book, *Body for Life*. I worked out that way for many years. As my knowledge grew, I formulated my own workout routine.

Probably the two most important elements in a workout are intensity (keep it high) and

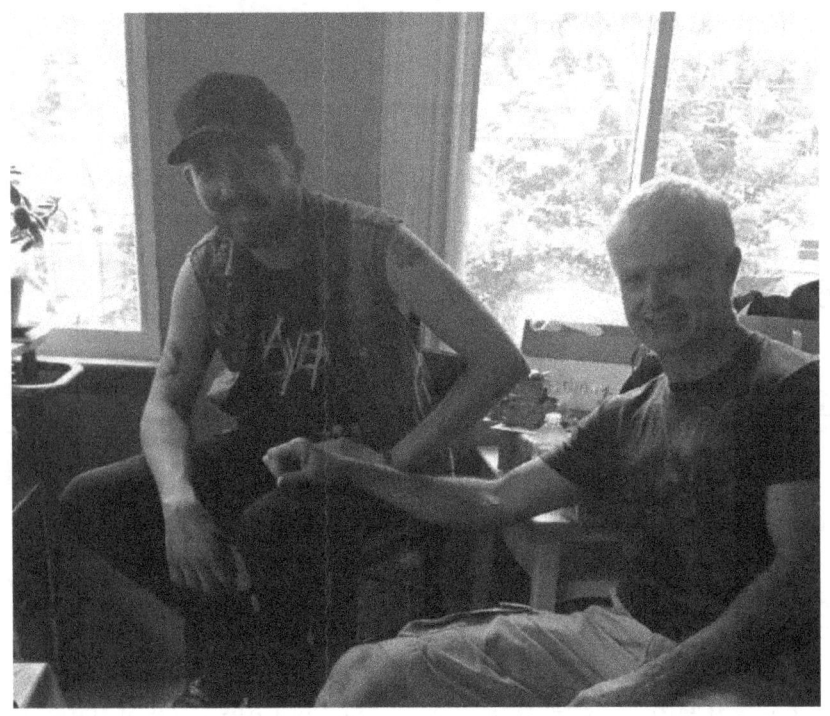

variety. Variety is important psychologically to keep things fresh and interesting but it's also important physiologically as well. The body is an extremely well designed machine that will find the path of least resistance. This is a good thing when doing an exercise because, more than likely, the correct way is the best way for your body to move. However, if any exercise is done consistently without changing some aspect of the routine, even the best exercise will fail to produce quality results after a while. Over the years, I have obtained (and am still obtaining) exercises for all the parts of the body. Utilizing this knowledge, I plug these exercises into the following routine. The constant changing of exercises and the manipulation of various aspects of the routine keeps it fresh and challenging.

I divide the month into two, two week cycles. During the first two weeks I do 3, 12 rep max sets. The last two weeks I do 4, 8 rep max sets. The first week I do chest, back and quads on Monday. On Tuesday, I do 30 – 40 minutes of cardio, abs and external rotator cuff exercises. Wednesday I do biceps, triceps, shoulders and abs. Thursday I do cardio and abs. Friday I do chest and back again and I also do hamstrings and calves. I take Saturday off and I do another ab routine and boxing on Sunday.

During the second week I repeat the above routine except that I switch things up doing arms and shoulders on Monday and Friday and chest and back on Wednesday. That way, I'm doing chest and back twice the first week and arms once. During the next week I do arms twice and chest and back once. The following two weeks, weeks three and four, I follow the same routine as above except that I do 8 rep max sets as described above.

I have read that the larger the muscle groups, the less times per week is needed to work them out. That is why I hit my legs basically once a week: fronts on Monday and backs on Friday. Then, during each two week cycle I hit the smaller muscle groups of the chest, arms and shoulders three times each. Abs, since they have a lot of endurance muscle fiber in them, can and need to be exercised more. So, each week I exercise them four times. I make a special effort to do cardio at least twice a week. However, in addition to that, my heart gets a good workout during my strength training because I utilize super sets (two exercises) and giant sets (three or more exercises) taking minimal rest between sets. Mind you, this is active rest, that is, while one muscle group is resting I'm exercising the opposing muscle group.

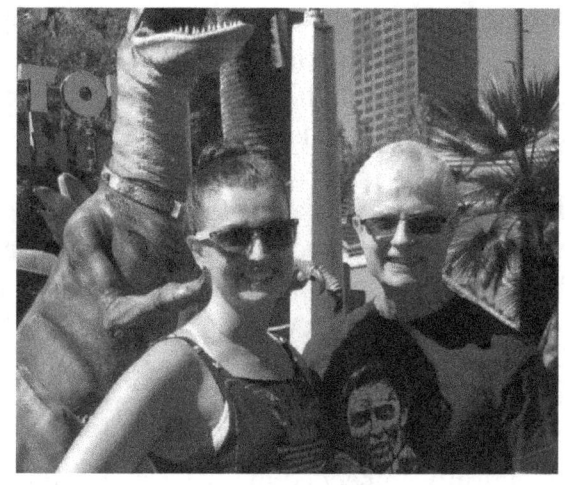

As I said, to do the same thing over and over will cause the body to plateau and not progress. This way of exercising, I've discovered, has built in changes. Just the way the training program is set up allows for a lot of changes merely in the schedule. With each session, a person can do different exercises.

Also, the way the exercises are put together and done is a change. My main way of exercising is opposing muscle groups: chest/back, biceps/ triceps, etc. However, once every two or three weeks I'll change things up by doing compound sets, that is, doing several exercises for the same muscle group back to back. This is a great plateau breaker.

What is your definition of passion? Heart? Success?

These three are as interconnected as a cocklebur in the hair of a dog (I just had to remove one from my dog's fur so this was fresh on my mind). If you are passionate about something in your heart, you will have success and the motivation to achieve that success.

Passion, simply put, is what drives us, or motivates us. It is what causes you to do what you do. It's why you get out of bed in the morning, put in a long day and go to bed late at night. It's what your mind keeps going back to. A person does a lot of things in the course of a day/week/year/lifetime, but it's what that person keeps returning to, whether in thought or in deed, is what that person is passionate about. We do what we are...and that, whatever it is, I feel is God given. How do you know what your passion is? Is it what you won't let go of? No, that's your desire. Your passion is what won't let go of you.

We in the west say heart. In one culture they say intestines. In another culture they say kidneys. Whether it's heart, intestines or kidneys, all these terms refer to the same thing: the essence of our being. It's the actual us; the actual you, the actual me, our respective spirits. These terms refer, in fact, to the core person. And once our passion gets into it, we will have...

Success! Success is achievement of our life's goals. Conquering, winning, overcoming obstacles, doing whatever it takes to accomplish what we've set our hearts to do. Passion embedded into the heart will not be distracted. It will not be defeated. We may stray or get discouraged but a passion truly seated in the heart will never be fully let go and the person will eventually return to it. We may get knocked down, but the passionate heart will not allow us to give up.

I, personally, have a goal I want to achieve. By having this goal firmly embedded in my heart, I will achieve it. And that is what transforms this goal into a lifestyle. Because this is so much a part of me (please refer back to the cocklebur in dog's hair illustration above), it has become more than just putting another notch in my belt or checking something else off of my to-do list. I am so focused on achieving this, that I spend every spare moment working on something that will eventually bring this into reality...and I've been working on it for years. When something is that important to you, that much a part of you, it is in many aspects, your life. However, and here's the really cool thing about being passionate about something, it's never a burden. In fact, it uplifts you and gives you purpose, your raison d'être.

What does Train to Live mean to you?

I see this as the flip side of the same coin we just discussed. If your passion is embedded in your heart and you are motivated by it to do whatever it takes to achieve it, this then becomes your lifestyle. But what if you don't feel well? What if everything hurts or you are so weak that just going from room to room, or up some stairs, or going to the grocery store, or (you fill in the blank) makes you want to lie down and take a two hour nap? Chances are, you're not going to get a lot accomplished achieving that lifetime goal you have set for yourself.

Live to train, or live to...whatever, is a common goal seen or heard everywhere. Really? Does a person actually live to train, or live to eat, or live to (again, you fill in the blank)? Unfortunately, some people do. These are the people who don't have a purpose for living, or are unfulfilled or experience that "hole in the soul". But, having that deeply embedded purpose for living in your heart gives you what you are living for. Now, the key is to make your body (read: dwelling place for your spirit, or heart) and mind as strong as you can and maintain that so that you can live, truly live, and accomplish that which you want to accomplish, that is...

Train to live. Train (do the right kind and amount of exercise and this includes eating the right amount, kind and quality of food, drinking the right amount of water, getting the right amount of sleep) to live (fulfilling that purpose, that thing which motivates you, and you live for, and gets you out of bed, and you keep returning to in your thoughts and deeds). Simply put, train so that you have the strength and stamina to do what you want/supposed/destined to do.

In the section before last, I discussed my workout. By no means is this *the* way to exercise and maintain your temple so that you can live your life, but it is definitely a way, and one that I have put to the test for years and can personally attest to its success.

Before we get into that though, let me ask you a question: How do you look in your genes? Or perhaps more accurately, how do you look with your genes? Although genetics has everything to do with how your body responds to exercise and should be at the very top of the list, it is mentioned rather seldom.

From the moment you are conceived your genetic blueprint was set getting various traits from both your mother's and father's side of their respective families. Genes determine everything from the color of your hair to whether you will have hair later in life. It determines eye color, body shape, body style, where fat

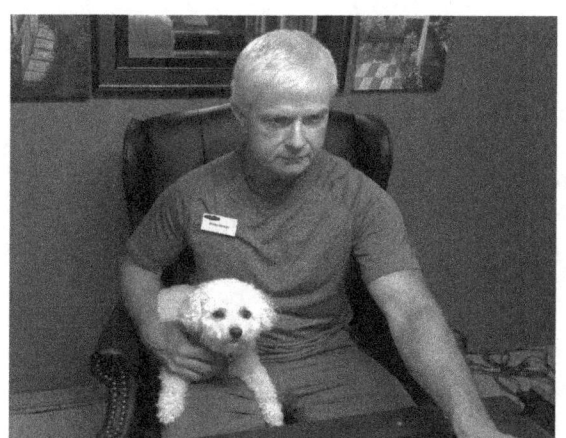

will be stored in your body, whether you will be a wiz at math or a wiz on the basketball court. It determines how much testosterone you will have (important for muscle building) and the ratio you have between the amount of muscle fiber type that gets bigger and develops (hypertrophy) and the muscle fiber type that allows you to run marathons (which will get stronger but not bigger, at least not as much as the other muscle fiber type just mentioned).

I can train ten different people, have them do the same workout, eat the same things, do everything in their training regimen the same and they will develop ten different ways because how a person's body responds to exercise and food intake is also determined by genetics. In other words, a greyhound will never be a mastiff and a mastiff will never be a greyhound.

I point this out to encourage you. Measure yourself with yourself, not someone else because...listen to me... that other person has different genetics than you do. Measuring your results with the results of someone else will only be frustrating. Therefore, a trainer can only promise to maximize your genetic potential.

Workouts that explain my style of training:

Chest, Back & Quads (front of the thighs)
With the exception of the quads, the chest and back, in this routine, will be done in super sets with little to no rest in between. To keep the intensity high, allow no more than 60 seconds rest between sets. I have a watch with a stop watch function on it. As soon as I'm finished with my chest exercise, I hit the button and proceed to do my back exercise. I usually have just enough time to make it back and do the next set of my chest exercise. I find this is a great way to do opposing muscle group super sets.

In regards to the weight, that is a matter of trying it out for yourself. Err on the side of caution. Start light and slow. When you begin working on a muscle you haven't trained during the current workout session, be sure to use light weights, watch your range of motion, form and speed. Do at least a couple of warm up sets before beginning your work sets. Listen to your body!!!!! Only when you feel your body is warmed up enough and it feels like you can do a heavier work load is the correct time for you to begin working that group of muscles.

Barbell bench press
Low Row
Incline, palm facing dumbbell bench press (keep continuous pressure on dumbbells
   pushing them together tightly during the entire motion of the press – this works the pecs
   simultaneously in both a fly and press motion: NOTE! This is an intense way to do a press
   and more than likely you will have to reduce the weight you normally use when doing an
   ordinary incline dumbbell press)

Lat pull down

Cable fly

Throat level pulls (adjust pulley so it's about chest high – attach rope attachment – grip rope with an underhand grip – pull rope back to upper chest or base of the neck – elbows are out to the side – abs are tight and squeeze shoulder blades together at the end of the movement)

Because we will be working the quads only once a week, we want to hit them hard. Therefore, we will be doing a compound giant set with them. This means we will be doing three exercises for the quads with no rest in between. We will workout the hamstrings and calves the same way on Friday. CAUTION! If you've never worked your muscles this way before, be careful! This is a very intense way to work your muscles. Rest as needed with the goal of doing all the exercises back to back without rest. After completing a set of all the exercises, rest for no more that 60 seconds before beginning the next set.

Squat
Leg press
Leg extensions

Cardio, Abs, External Rotator Cuff

It has been found that the most beneficial way to exercise your heart muscle is to do cardio exercises varying the intensity during each workout. This can be done in a couple of ways; interval training and cross training.

Interval training is usually done using one mode of exercise and varying the intensity. For example, if you exercise on a treadmill, you can change the intensity by increasing the incline or the speed. Alternate periods of lower intensity with periods of higher intensity such as walking briskly for a minute and then running for a minute. Most machines have built in programs you may use. These are preset ways of interval training. However, be careful when using these preset programs and make sure you are able to do them without injuring yourself.

Cross training is done utilizing more than one mode of exercise (I use this method because, I admit, when it comes to cardio I have ADD). For example, for a 30 minute cardio routine, I will sometimes use a treadmill, elliptical and a climb stairs (not a stair stepper machine, actual stairs – where I work I have the advantage of being in an 18 story building so I put the stairs to good use). For five minutes, I power walk on the treadmill (sometimes I combine interval and cross training by power walking for a minute and then running for a minute). Then I switch and do five minutes on the elliptical. Finally, I complete my first round by climbing stairs for five minutes. I do that all again for a set of 30 minutes.

This is just an example. You can do any kind of cardio exercise or use any kind of cardio equipment: walking/running outside, bicycling, roller blading, swimming, jumping rope, etc. The main thing is to keep your heart challenged. Using the interval method you change the way your heart beats by varying the intensity. Using the cross training method you change the way your heart beats by utilizing different exercises – each of those exercises will cause your body to work in a slightly different way and therefore affect your heart rate accordingly.

Abs and core are used synonymously. However, abs are your actual abdominal muscles whereas your core is comprised of all of the muscles in your torso. So, your abs are part of your core but it's important to exercise your entire core including your abs, for good posture, fighting back pain, stability and strength (because the core is the foundation of the human body, we get our strength from it just as the superstructure of a building gets its strength from its foundation), and etc. Speaking of the abs part of your core, because there are so many muscles which make up the abdominal structure, it is best to hit them from all directions – and we will do just that.

The external rotator cuff muscles are probably one of the weakest muscles in the body, and for good reason. Activities of daily living and exercises we do in the gym, for the most part, involve an inward rotation of the shoulder and our arm coming in towards the midline of the body (adduction). So our internal rotators are naturally strong. Weak external rotators lies at the base of shoulder injury, back injury and, related to that, the C shape that a lot of people who work desk jobs get. This C shape (battling this is also tied in with good ab and core strength) leads to more problems. We are designed to stand and sit erect. When we slump, or go into that C shape, our lungs can't fill with oxygen and our heart can't work as well which causes our muscles and organs not to get the quality and quantity of oxygen and blood they need for maximum performance. So, the more we can exercise this muscle group, the better we can counteract what life puts upon us and, what we put upon ourselves.

Cardio
Treadmill (1% incline, 5 minutes, speed – brisk walk; for added intensity, alternate one
        minute walking with one minute of running)
Elliptical (5-10 resistance, 5 minutes)
Stairs (5 minutes on actual stairs or stair master)
Repeat above routine once for 30 minutes, twice for 45 minutes, etc.

Abs

The abdominal muscles are torso muscles. Remember, the torso extends from your shoulders to your hips. In order to activate these muscles you need to get your torso involved in the movement.

Ab sling reverse crunch (10-25 reps, focus on pulling the hips up towards the ribs – legs bent, easier; legs straight, more challenging)
Wood chop (10-25 reps)
Ball crunch (10-25 reps, hold a weight on chest or above it for an extra challenge)
Roll outs on a physio ball (10-20 reps)
Repeat above routine 3 times if maxing out at 10-15 reps; 2 times if maxing out at 16 or more reps.

External shoulder rotators

Use a cable machine or tubing intense enough to fatigue muscles between 10-12 reps. Do 3 sets of each exercise. Rest 30 seconds between each set. One side, then the other is one set.

Mid (a little higher than your navel) cable or mid tube attachment – Grab handle, bend elbow 90°, keep elbow at side (holding a rolled up towel at your side with your elbow helps keep arm in position). Keep forearm parallel to floor. Begin with forearm just off of torso, rotate out as far as you can maintaining good form. Return to starting position and repeat.

High (about head high) cable or high tube attachment – Grab handle, bend elbow 90°, raise upper arm so that it is parallel to the floor. Maintaining the 90° bend in the elbow, starting position is with the forearm also parallel to the floor. Rotate forearm 90° back until forearm is perpendicular to the floor. Return to starting position and repeat.

Low (lowest cable setting or anchored just above the floor) cable or low tube attachment - Grab handle. Arm is technically straight with a slight bend at the elbow. Allow arm to go from shoulder to opposite hip across torso at about a 45° angle. Palm faces body at the starting position. Engage abs and maintaining arm position, pull handle in an arcing motion 180° from starting position so that the arm is extended 45° off of shoulder. Palm is now facing away from body. Return to starting position and repeat.

Biceps, Triceps, Shoulders, Abs
Incline spider curl
Close grip barbell press

Barbell curl
Triceps push down

Incline hammer curl
Arnolds

Barbell shrugs
Standing lateral raise

Captain's chair
Ab sling side crunch (one side at a time or alternate sides)
Ab wheel

Cardio, Abs
Outside power walk/run (Running on actual ground rather than on a treadmill, is much the same as climbing actual stairs as opposed to using a stair climbing machine. On both you are pushing your body weight against gravity therefore giving you more resistance and therefore giving you a more intense workout. Alternate one minute of walking as hard and fast as you can with one minute of running. Continue this walk/run pattern for 30 to 40 minutes)

Ab sling toes to the bar (remember, focus on pulling your hips up to actually contract the abdominal muscles. Control the lowering of the legs for a good, eccentric contraction)
Russian twists (hold onto a dumbbell or weight plate for added intensity)
Ab wheel

Chest, Back , Hamstrings, Calves
Dips (assisted dip machine, body weight or weighted depending on desired intensity)
T-bar row

Incline barbell bench press
Pull-ups (assisted pull-up machine, body weight or weighted depending on desired intensity)

Pec deck fly
Pec deck reverse fly

Romanian (straight leg) *dead lift*
Hamstring curls
Calf raises (use a machine designed for this, or a leg press with the heels hanging over the bottom of the

foot plate, or single legs holding a dumbbell with feet on a step or elevated
    object allowing the heels to hang lower than the toes. These all get the superficial calf muscle, the gastrocnemius with assistance from the deep calf muscle, the soleus. If you have access to a seated calf machine, which emphasizes the soleus, utilize this as well either on the same day you work the gastrocnemius or alternating weeks between the gastrocnemius and soleus)

Remember, the next week we switch, working out arms and shoulders twice, on Monday and Friday, and chest and back once, on Wednesday. Below is an additional workout for the arms, shoulders and abs.

Biceps, Triceps, Shoulders, Abs   (Second Workout)
Standing dumbbell curl with forearm rotation (begin with arms hanging down at sides with
    palms facing legs. When the dumbbells clear the legs rotate the forearm so at the end of
    the motion the palms face the shoulders)
Lying dumbbell triceps extensions

Strongman (or Strongwoman – gotta be PC you know) curls (Set the pulleys at their highest setting on a cable machine. Use the handle attachments. Grab the handles and stand in the middle of the pulleys. With your chest up, shoulder back and down and pulling your navel in towards your spine creating a tight core, position your arms so that the upper part of your arms are parallel to the floor. Extend your arms and keeping everything still, except the forearms, flex your elbows contracting your biceps bringing your fists in towards your head. At the maximum point of the movement, pause for a second, squeeze the biceps then return to the starting position and repeat)
Underhand grip triceps extension (utilizing a curl or straight bar attachment attached to a high pulley)

Low cable hammer curl **(utilizing the rope attachment attached to a low pulley)**
Overhead, knuckles out shoulder press

Standing lateral raise (leaning slightly forward at the hip and keeping back straight and abs tight)
Low cable front raise (utilizing the V-bar attachment attached to a low pulley pulling it up between the legs. Keep arms relatively straight and abs tight)

Captain's chair (bent or straight leg)
Torso twists (like wood chops mentioned above except the pulley is positioned just below chest level on a cable machine. Arms are kept straight out and remain relatively parallel to the floor. Pull navel in towards spine creating a tight core and focus on rotating the torso so that the arms just come along for the ride 180° away from the pulley. Pause for a second then return to the starting position and repeat)
High cable weighted crunches (using either the rope attachment or ab slings attached to the pulley at the

highest position on a cable machine, kneel down facing away from the pulley. Grasping the rope, or placing elbows in the ab slings, pull one or the other down on either side of your head resting hands or elbows on the chest. Lean forward from the knees keeping body straight from the knees to the ears. Tighten core and flex abs just below the point where the ribs come together below the chest. Squeeze abs at the apex of the movement for a second, return to starting position and repeat)

Plank (set a time to hold the plank and go for that goal; a few seconds, a minute, two, etc. This can be the conventional forearm/toes plank, extended arms plank, or dynamic plank raising the arms and legs in certain patterns)

Compound Workout Examples

These will give you an idea of what to do on those plateau breaker weeks addressed above. Remember, these are done back to back, in a group, with no rest in between the exercises. That's the goal. When starting out, rest as needed. Take your time, be careful and listen to your body. When you have achieved the "no rest in between exercises" status, rest for 30 to 60 seconds between group sets.

Chest
Dumbbell bench press
Incline barbell press
Cable fly

Back
Low row
Lat pull down
Reverse pec deck fly

Biceps

Incline dumbbell spider curls
Standing dumbbell curls
Seated incline dumbbell hammer curls

Triceps

Standing double dumbbell kick-backs
Incline lying dumbbell triceps extensions
Lying dumbbell triceps extensions

Shoulders

Lateral raise
Upright row
Dumbbell overhead shoulder press

At the end of your workout, stretching is recommended. Your muscles are warm and more supple so you can get a better stretch. Some schools of thought promote stretching to avoid blood pooling and to remove lactic acid from worked muscles. One thing is for certain, stretching after every workout will allow you to move easier and more freely. Bruce Lee and one of his main students, Danny Inosanto, were walking along Venice Beach, California one time. Danny was amazed at the huge body builders working out there. Bruce patiently looked at them, turned to Danny and said, "Yes, but can they use that strength?" Good point! We've trained to be stronger. Now, let's finish with some stretching so that we can "use" it.

Stretching can be best done utilizing static stretching, foam rolling or both. With a static stretch, get into a position to stretch a certain muscle, or muscle groups. It has been suggested to hold the stretch for at least 10 seconds all the way up to 30 seconds. But, as was brought out before, listen to your body.
To maximize the effect of the stretch and to benefit most from it, you need to override your body's stretch reflex. Once you get into a stretch position you will feel the muscle tighten. That's normal. It's your body's reaction to the stretch preventing the muscle from becoming injured. That's why you want to hold the stretch until you feel the muscle relax. It's like telling your body, "It's OK. I know what I'm doing and not going to hurt you." One doctor describes it as "feeling the melt". Continue with your other muscles in the same way.

Foam rolling is another method of stretching that can be used as an alternative or complement to static stretching. There is a milky, fibrous material surrounding all muscles called fascia. Foam rolling causes myo-fascial release. It's the same thing you receive when you get a deep tissue massage (except it won't cost you $100). As you roll the foam roller over your muscles you will feel what I refer to as "wince" spots. These are spots on the muscle which are extremely tight and when you roll over them you just may "wince" with a little pain. Again, this is normal and the more you do it, the less winces you will receive. Whichever method you choose is fine, but be sure to stretch out after your workout in some manner.

My favorite quotes:

I really enjoy quotes. They can take a complicated idea, theory, or philosophy and simplify it in such a way so that you can remember it. Here are a few of my favorites.

"The good is the enemy of the best."   Oswald Chambers

"Whether you think you can, or you think you can't--you're right."   Henry Ford

"If you want to hit the tops of the trees, aim for the moon."   Bruce Lee

"Life experience will either make you better or it will make you bitter."   T. D. Jakes

"The graveyard is the richest place on earth, because it is here that you will find all the hopes and dreams that were never fulfilled, the books that were never written, the songs that were never sung, the inventions that were never shared, the cures that were never discovered, all because someone was too afraid to take that first step, keep with the problem, or determined to carry out their dream."
   Les Brown

"When there is no enemy within, the enemies outside cannot hurt you."   African Proverb

And last but definitely not least, my all time favorite quote...

"Do unto others as you would have them do unto you."
Jesus

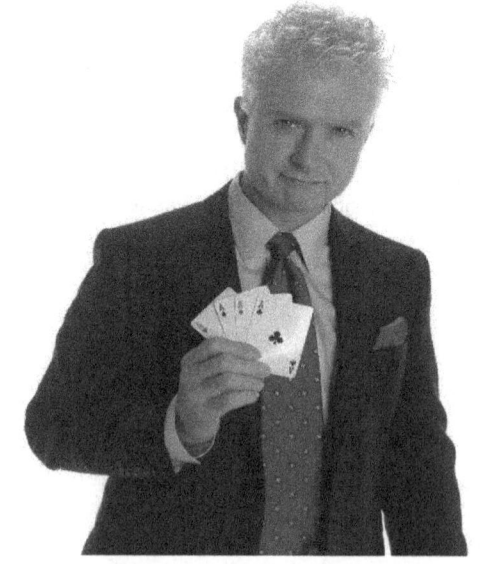

To paraphrase this last one in the modern vernacular, "**Treat others the way you want to be treated**." Yeah, yeah, we all know this one. It's the Golden Rule, right? I've been hearing this since I was a kid. Yes, we may have heard it, and know it by heart, but have you really ever considered the deep implications of this very "simple" command? Think about it. If everyone actually practiced this every day, we could get rid of laws, police, judges, courts, the military, charitable organizations and perhaps even banks and lending institutions. Have I gone too far? Not really.

If, and I know this is a huge if, however, if everyone actually carried this out, with everyone, every day, all the things listed above could indeed take place. *#mindblown*

Client Testimony:
-Janna Pearman-Jacob

I am a runner and have been going to Forrest for several years. I started because a friend recommended I try strength training with a personal trainer to balance out my running. I tried it and found I really liked it. I have never done any strength training before and having a trainer helped me focus on my specific goals and not get injured. I have stuck with it because I like the results – my energy level and how I look in my clothes!

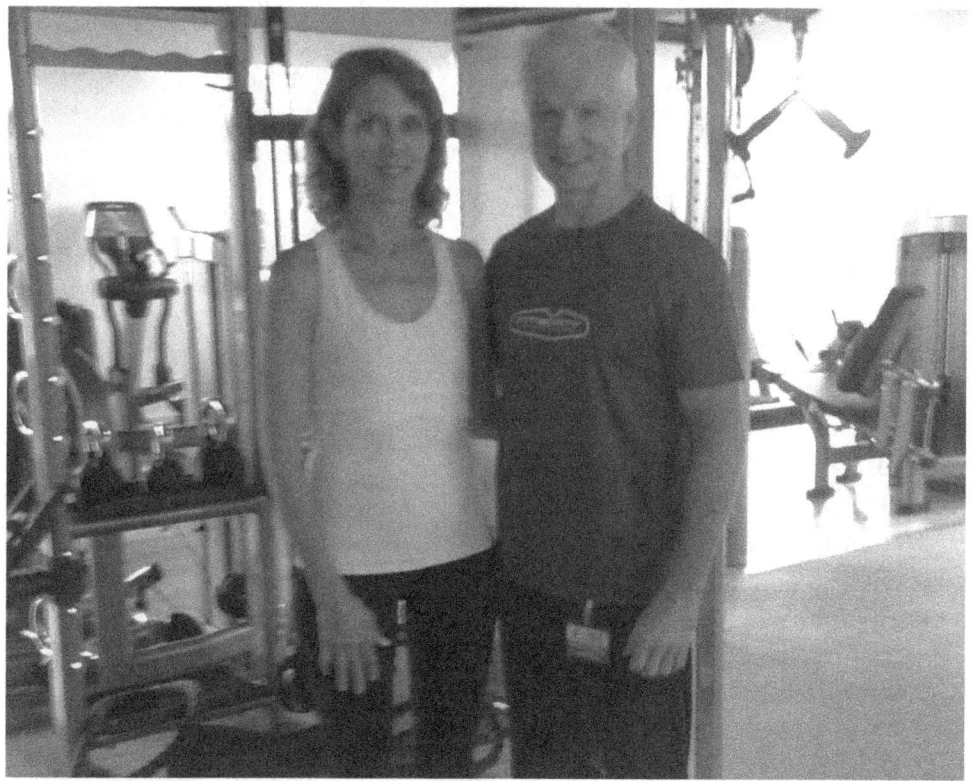

Client Testimony:
-Michelle Murray

I have been working out with integrity training systems for about nine months now and I feel stronger than ever before. I just decided I needed a personal trainer when I just lacked the motivation to work out. I have tried various exercise programs including title boxing which I enjoy but it was primarily cardio and I have been reading a lot about the importance of strength training as you age and maintaining flexibility. So I decided to reach out to a trainer that I had worked out with nearly 15 years ago, Forrest Boston. Thankfully his cell phone number has not changed so I was able to connect with him and get on his schedule. One of the things I love about working out with Forrest is that he is so highly educated on physical fitness. He doesn't just explain how to do an exercise with good form he explains the physiological reasons why this exercise works and it always makes perfect sense to me. He's a great teacher and motivator and he's very positive never ever negative. After several months of working out with Forrest twice a week I was also introduced to Debbie and I was referred to her for a nutrition plan because I was experiencing a lot of vertigo and the doctors could not figure out what was wrong. I was also having tremendous joint pain and had been tested for some immune disorders that tended to run in my family. Thankfully all of those test turned out negative but I was still left with no help and I was left with sheer exhaustion, ringing in my ears, and severe vertigo to the point where I would work during the day and come home about o'clock and sleep until six. So with one meeting from Debbie she put me on a really strict diet to reduce any inflammation causing foods in my diet and histamine causing foods and she also recognizes instantly that I was off-balance and it was likely due to a cranial structure and not any internal biological causes. So she referred me to an outstanding therapist and with just one half-hour session was able to rid me of the ringing in my ears and after a few short sessions she was able to cure the vertigo that I was experiencing. Between these three folks working with in sync at Integrity I felt like my life has changed. I can't tell you how much weight I've lost because I avoid scales but I can say that my size 4 and 6 clothes fit a heck of a lot better than they did nine months ago and more importantly I feel healthier and much, much stronger and just overall better physically fit!

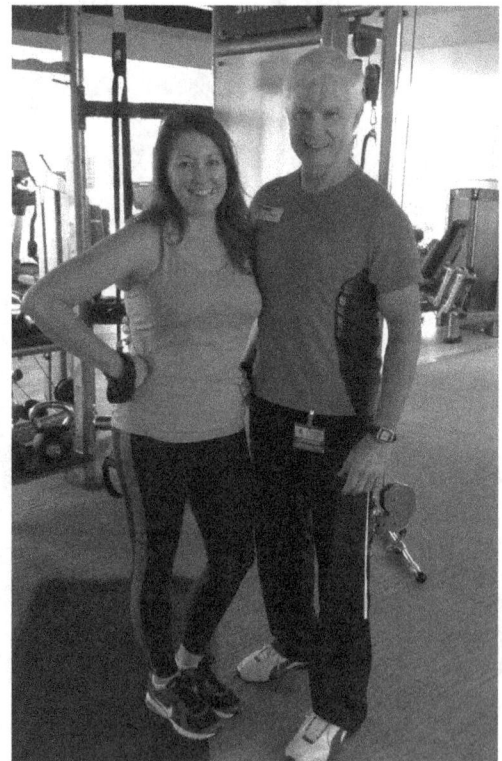

Why should you choose Integrity?

Merriam-Webster defines "integrity" as 1) the quality of being honest and fair and 2) the state of being complete or whole, undivided. This is Integrity Training Systems. However, this term is more than just the name of the company. Integrity is a term which describes the quality of the individuals who work for this company as well as the quality of the product which this company provides.

I've heard it said that a boss demands, but a leader leads – they get into the trenches with the employees and lead by example. This is exactly what the founder of Integrity Training Systems, Debbie Portell, does. She sets ultra high standards for herself and her employees, and each and every day she exemplifies this, asking only from her staff that which she does herself, first.

With a leader like this, it's no mistake that these high standards and qualities are in all the employees of Integrity. All trainers at Integrity carry certifications from nationally recognized certifying agencies. Being thoroughly educated in exercise science, kinesiology, anatomy, physiology, nutrition, as well as special needs for people who have certain musculoskeletal injuries, disease and other medical conditions, we work with our clients to maximize their genetic potential. We continue to educate ourselves on the latest research in exercise science so we remain at the cutting edge, always improving, striving for perfection, to make our clients the absolute best they can be.

But, beyond this, we care. There are no rubber stamp, gloss-over sessions here. We speak with you, we listen to you and hear your needs, mentally, physically, socially, emotionally and spiritually, and do whatever we can to help you. You are not a meal ticket to us. Yes, we are a business and we strive to grow, but we recognize that our business is helping people, just like you, doing whatever it takes and doing whatever we can to help you. Sometimes this may even mean that we refer you to a professional outside of our organization acknowledging that this person will be able to help you even more. But together, with God's help, we make a team to serve you and meet your needs.

Of course, these are mere words. So, put us to the test. Take us for a test drive. Come and get to know us. We will give you a free assessment and maybe even a free session. See for yourself that we want to, and can, help you.

What made you a trainer?
Mike Stout

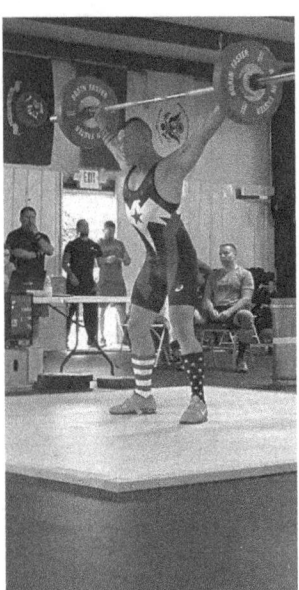

I first became a trainer because I enjoyed working out and seeing my own transformation from exercise. I liked how I looked but more importantly, how I felt. I wanted to share this with as many people as I could so that they would be able to achieve the same results and the same feelings I went through.

I am a trainer because I have a passion for helping people. It is such a rewarding feeling watching the emotions people have when they hit a goal that is important to them. I feel a great sense of accomplishment when they are able to tell me how much better they feel, physically and mentally.

I quickly learned that not everyone that comes in to see me wants to have a killer workout. Most of my clients were dealing with aches and pains and wanted to have them resolved. That is when I started educating myself on injuries, stretching, and corrective exercises. I absolutely get excited and pumped if a client hits a big lift that they have been working towards, but when I have a client tell me that they can go up and down the stairs with out getting out of breath and not having pain in their there knees or back, that is the real accomplishment that makes me happy.

What inspires you to wake up each day and live your passion each day? My clients inspire me to set an example and keep sharing the ever growing knowledge that I have on health and fitness. I want all of my clients to know the difference of good form versus bad form, not just what it looks like but what it feels like so they can correct it on their own as well as understanding why they need to be in a certain position and how it benefits them.

What are your strengths?

My strengths include corrective exercises and mobility, calisthenics, and barbell training (power lifting, weightlifting)

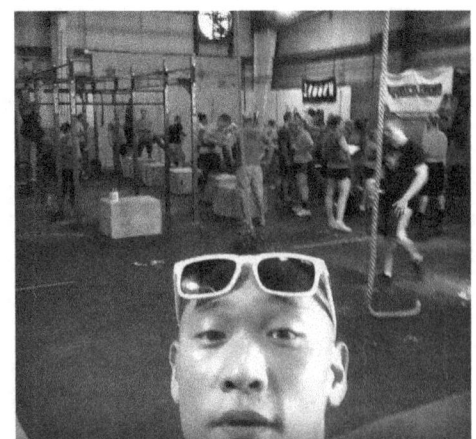

Weaknesses?

My weaknesses include nutrition information. I always felt like I had great guidelines for clients to follow and general information. The amount of detail that Debbie goes into with her nutrition program makes me realize that I still have a vast amount of information to learn and understand in order to better myself as a trainer and improve my clients as well.

My current focus is on competitive weightlifting (olympic movements; snatch, clean and jerk) and my goals are for my total to exceed 200 kilograms (440 pounds) by next years competition.

What is your philosophy on nutrition?

I commonly tell my clients that they should eat to live and not live to eat. Focus more on what your body needs and less on what tastes good. Many people will over eat and make portions larger because something tastes good. They increase the amount of calories they take in but do not increase activity levels to match. We have to be conscious and aware of everything that we eat or drink, especially if we are working towards a change in body composition. I have talked with many people trying to lose weight that will unnecessarily eat snacks and sweets but they do not understand why they can not lose weight.

I mostly eat chicken, eggs, salmon, spinach, and rice. I can eat the same thing and not get bored with it and with these options I can cook a large amount at the same time.

Do you take supplements?

Yes! Magnesium, for muscle cramps. Glutamine, to help repair muscle and prevent breakdown. Citrulline, to help reduce muscular fatigue. Bela Alanine and Creatine to help promote muscular endurance.

What is your workout schedule & why?

Mostly my workout schedule is based on recovery. Depending on where my schedule is at for competition, I will work in squat, deadlift, and olympic variations 3-5 times per week and work in auxiliary movements, upper body, and mobility exercises throughout the rest of the week. I seem to always have a "sore" feeling, so when I base my schedule on recovery it is mostly making sure that I have the mobility to perform the movements safely. Even "rest" days should have time spent actively recovering or working on technique.

What is your definition of passion? Heart? Success?

Passion is something that drives you to be the best no matter how many failed attempts or obstacles get in your way. Your passion is something that you enjoy doing and does not feel like a chore.

Heart is doing what you believe is right and not letting anything stop you.

Success is accomplishing something important to you. I do not believe that success is not measured in money or titles but in actions.

How do you stay motivated to make this a lifestyle and not a goal?

I grew up without any knowledge of exercise or nutrition. I quickly became overweight and struggled with confidence. I did not like how I looked or how I felt but I did not know how to work towards changing my body composition. My ultimate goal was to make it a lifestyle. Once I got in "good shape" I wanted to maintain that and once I became a trainer I wanted to set an example for my clients. If I could go from eating fries, nachos, and ice cream; to eating chicken, salmon, and spinach; I certainly could inspire my clients to do the same.

What does Train to Live mean to you?

To me, Train to Live means just that. Train for life. Train your body to be able to squat, run, and jump. If not to survive the zombie apocalypse then to be able to play with your kids instead of sitting on a bench watching from the sidelines or to go on vacation and see all of the sites without any restriction due to physical strength.

Why should you choose Integrity?

People should choose Integrity because of the friendly and fun atmosphere paired with knowledgable and professional trainers.

Workouts that explain my style of training:

Back
3 Rounds
10 Deadlift Row combination
15 Assisted Pull Ups
20 cable Cross Low Row
20 Bent Over Reverse Fly

4 Rounds
15 Cable Pronated High Row
15 Cable Supinated Low Row
5 Heavy Lat Pull
15 Light Lat Pull

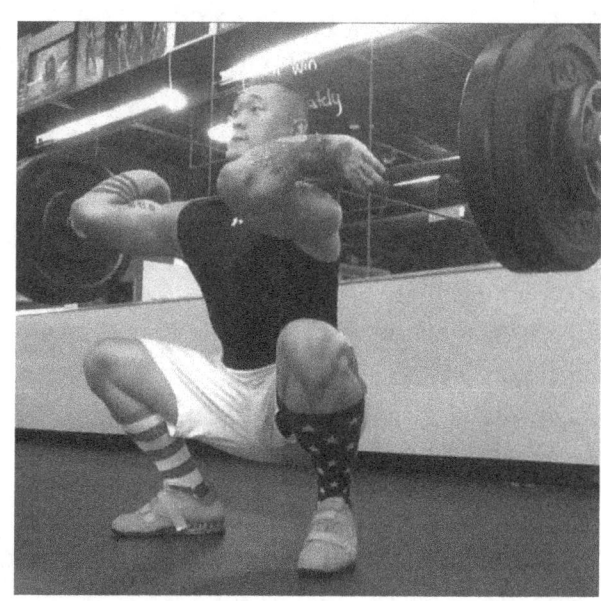

3 Rounds
10 Dumbbell Row (each arm)
20 Back Extension
15 Band Pull Aparts
20 Seated Neutral Grip Row

Shoulders
4 Rounds
10 Pronated Press
10 Neutral Press
20 Lateral Raises
20 Front Raises

3 Rounds
50 Battle Rope Slams
10 Inchworms
20 Plank Ups
20 Hand Walk Overs from Box

3 Rounds
15 Upright Rows
20 Behind the Neck Press or Military Press
20 Alternating Seated Shoulder Press

Legs
3 Rounds
15 each Single Leg-Leg Press
Heavy Sled pull/push
10 Swing Squat
20 Leg Extension
20 Leg Curl

3 Rounds
15 Stiff Leg Deadlift
20 Dumbbell Walking Lunges
15 Goblet Squat

15 Stability Ball Leg Curls
10 Single Leg Lunges

3 Rounds
10 each Dumbbell Step Ups
20 Squat Pulses
10 Jump Squats
10 each Lunge Kicks

Cardio
100 Jump Rope
5 minutes on a station with 30 seconds high intensity/60 seconds low intensity
Stair Master - Elliptical - Treadmill- Rower - Versa Climber - Bike
100 Jump Rope
60 Seconds on a station
Burps - Ball Slam - Mountain Climbers - Battle Rope - Jumping Jacks - Box Jumps
100 Jumper Rope

Core
3 Rounds
30 Toe Touches
25 V-sit Crunches
20 Plank Twists
15 Leg Lift with Hip Raise
10 V-Ups

2 Rounds
20 each Side Plank Pulses
40 Penguins
15 each Side Plank Pulses
30 Penguins
10 each Side Plank Pulses
20 Penguins

3 Rounds
10 Windshield Wipers
20 each Single Leg Straight Arm Plank Hops
20 Sit Ups
20 Mountain Climbers

Mobility
Improving Squat Positioning
Foam Roll: Quads, Inner/Outer Thigh, Hamstrings, Calves
Ball Roll: Glutes Pecs, Lats, Deltoids
Stretch: Pecs, Lats, Hip Flexors, Hamstrings, Glutes, Calves
Strengthen: Glutes/Abductors (Hip Bridge, Banded Side Steps, Back (Row, Lat Pull, Back Extension)

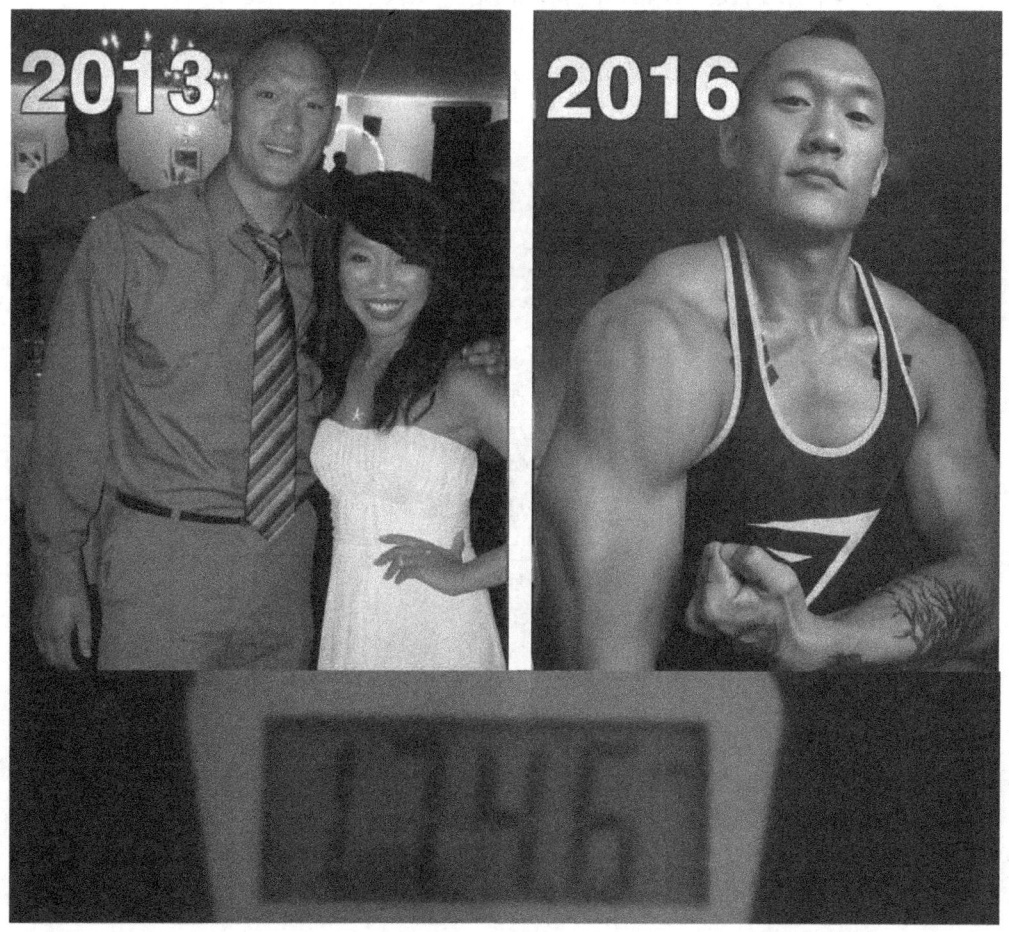

My favorite quotes:

"The body achieves what the mind believes"

"Challenge brings change"

"Commit to be fit"

"Work hard in silence and let success be your noise"

"It's what you do in the dark that puts you in the light"

"Set your bar high, be kind and do more of what makes you stronger"

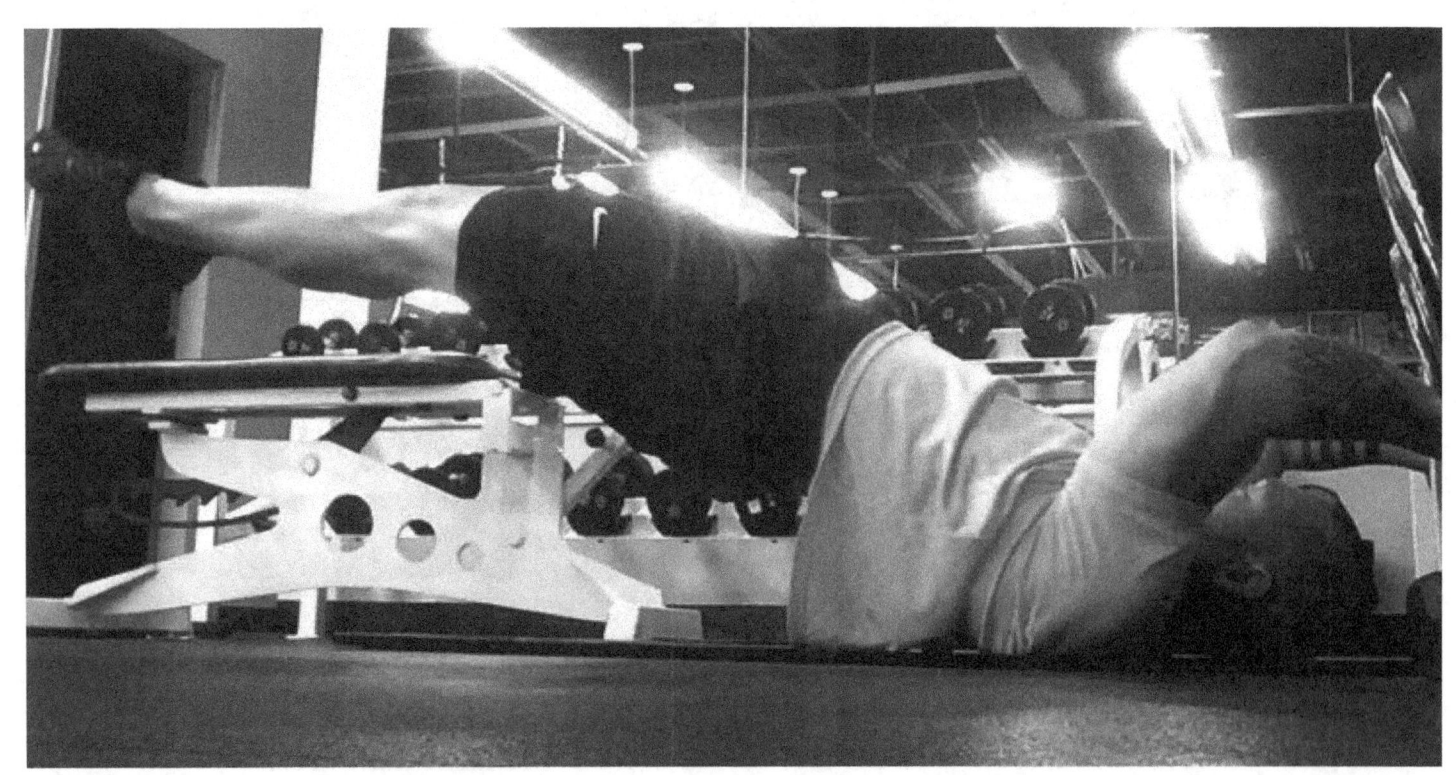

Client Testimony:
-Brian Bauer

I knew this day was coming and today it was finally here. I just received the results of my physical and many of the numbers were bad. Blood pressure 139/98, cholesterol 261, 2 elevated enzymes on my liver, and my weight is at an all time high of 212 pounds. The pizzas, chips, fast food, and beer had caught up to me. My doctor said that I would have to go on high blood pressure and cholesterol medication or make some serious lifestyle changes. I did not want to go on medication. The last thing I wanted to do was to sit down at the beginning of every week and sort medications into a weekly pill dispenser.

I had listened to the Healthy Living radio show on occasion when I was in the car on Sunday afternoons. I was impressed with what I had heard so I went to the Integrity Training Group web site and filled out the contact form. Later that same day Debbie sent me back some information on how to get started and the process to regain my health had begun.

My first meeting with Debbie was an exchange of information. I explained to her what my health conditions and goals were and she wrote out a meal plan specifically designed to address those needs. I conveyed to her that one of my main health enemies was time. Since I work long hours Debbie told me that planning and preparing meals in advance would be critical to my success. With that in mind, every Sunday I prepared enough chicken, salmon, and vegetables for the week. Then, each day before I left for work I'd fill a cooler with my daily meals, grab a gallon jug of water, and head out the door. Two and a half weeks later before my first follow up meeting I stepped on the scale. I had lost 13 pounds! Debbie would continue to make adjustments to my food at each follow up meeting. The weight continued to fall off and my waist continued to shrink. Now that my food was on track I wanted to start exercising again. Debbie put me in contact with one of her personal trainers - Mike Stout.

The purpose of my first meeting with Mike was to assess my physical imbalances and determine my overall physical condition. I had plenty of imbalances and was not in very good physical shape either. I began working out with Mike two times a week. Mike's main concern was to give me a great workout that corrected my imbalances that was also injury free. His knowledge seemed endless. Foam rolling, stretching, free weights, and the weight machines were explained in great detail. He would teach me the proper form for each exercise and would not have me do certain movements until my body was absolutely ready for it. My strength and stamina increased with each session.

The care and concern for my health from both Debbie and Mike is truly genuine. They really want to heal me. Debbie focused mainly on the nutrition while Mike focused on the strengthening and aligning of my body. The results have been extreme. My blood pressure has dropped to 111/73. I have lost 41 pounds and 7 inches off my waist. I can't wait for my next doctor's appointment.

I have recently completed the 3 month nutrition program with Debbie but continue to work out with Mike once a week. I'd like to thank my wife Tracie, along with my friends and family for all of their support. I have no doubt that I can take the knowledge taught to me from Integrity Training Systems and continue to live a healthy lifestyle. Now if I could only master that squat technique.

Client Testimony:
-Jim Light

Having just been released from spinal surgery, I looked for the perfect rehab. I found it to be a company named Integrity. I was assigned a therapist named Mike Stout, and couldn't have been happier with the choice. All post op problems are being addressed and I am improving rapidly.

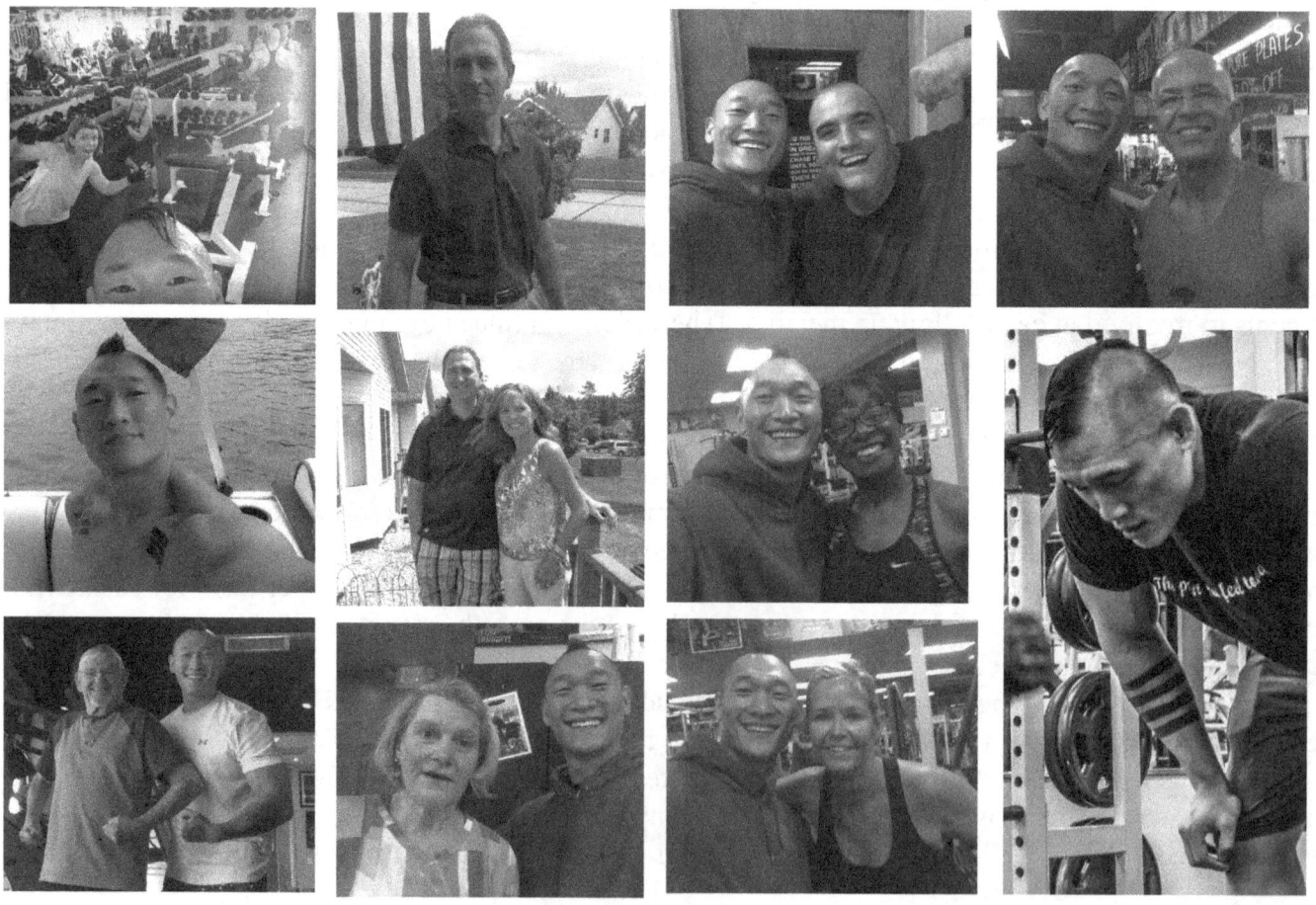

What made you a trainer?
Mike Lumia

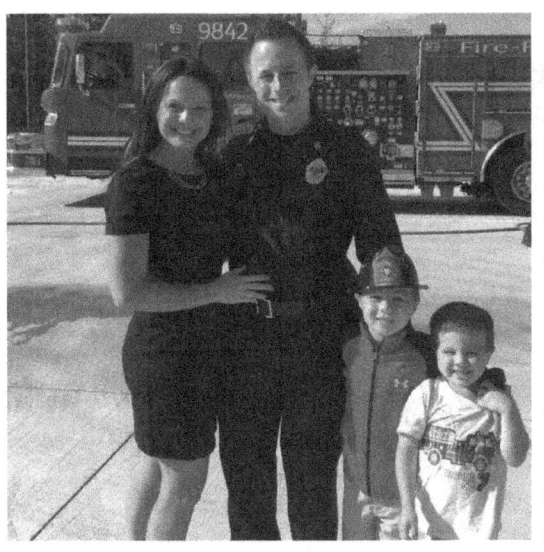

A lot of things made me a trainer starting with always being involved in sports mainly wrestling and BJJ/MMA. I started getting more interested in to the fitness sides of these sports. I started having other people ask me for advice on weight loss & will I help them to get motivated to workout. I was constantly in the gym working out trying new exercises to see what would end up changing my body. I finally decided to get certified through NASM, which is a great accomplishment but in my opinion after this I still wasn't a trainer. I knew I needed more so I went out to look for more training. I had met with other gyms who were ready to put me out on the floor just because of the certification I had, but I declined their offer. I meet with Integrity and they recommended I do 6 sessions with every trainer they have. I knew it was a lot to take on but believed that the best training I was looking for was here. I learned so much from every trainer here from workouts, exercises, nutrition, and be the best version of myself. Everyone at Integrity made and continues to make me a better trainer.

There are many reasons why I became a trainer which makes it hard to explain. I want to inspire people. I want someone to look at me and say "because of you I didn't give up." I was working out with one of my co-workers at the fire department. He was saying all morning how he wanted me to come up with a workout for him and motivate him to do it. So I did, I created him a workout and pushed him through it. At the end he was tired, sweating, & out of breath. He looked at me and said "Thanks man, that was a great workout there is no way I could of done it without you." That's why I am a trainer.

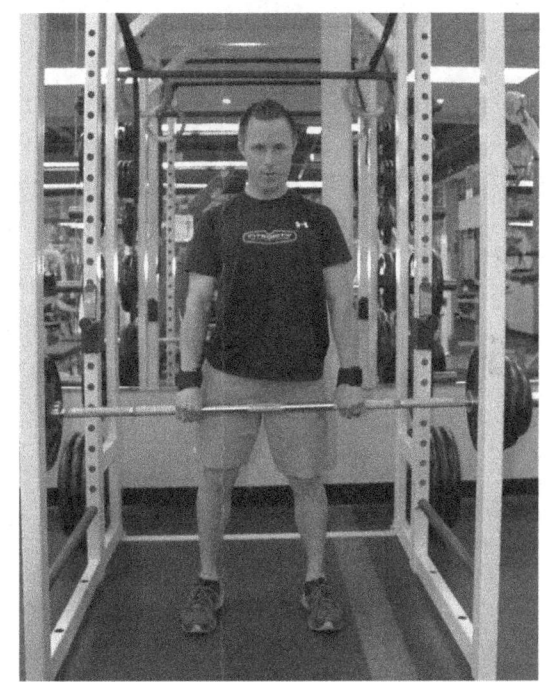

What inspires you to wake up each day and live your passion each day?

"We Rise By Lifting Others". The feeling I get when my clients get taken off their blood pressure medication, lose/gain weight, tone up, when they tell me that I never would of pushed myself like this if you weren't here. It's the lives I can change every day for kids to seniors. I feed off of that feeling every day to help them and others.

What are your strengths?

I'm very goal driven, so when a goal or challenge is set for someone or myself. I will do whatever it takes to make it happen. I don't ever want to look back and think that one time I gave 95% instead of giving 100% was the reason I or I didn't reach goal.

Weaknesses?

Sometimes my weaknesses can also come from my strengths. I'm very passionate & goal driven for others to succeed I put a lot of pressure on myself of what I can do differently or better for them. I tend to neglect things outside of the gym because I'm so focused on them succeeding. I need to learn how to balance booth.

What has your focus and what are your goals?

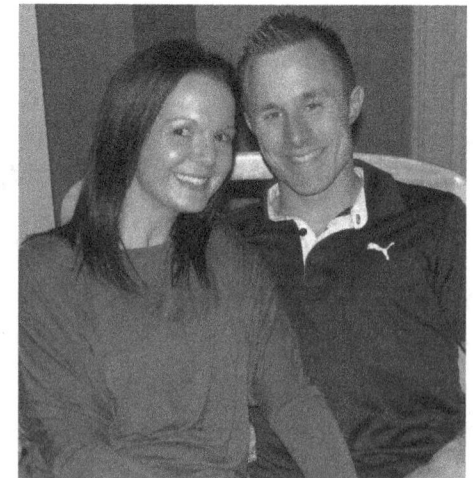

Be the best firefighter I can be. Be the best trainer I can be.
Be the best friend I can be. Be the best family man I can be.
Be the best version of me I can be.

What is your philosophy on nutrition?

I definitely have learned a lot about nutrition since training at Integrity. I've not only seen food help weight control but help clients get off of their Rx, control body swelling, bloating, inflammation,. and more. Everyone's body reacts to food differently so it's not all about counting calories, points, and macros. It's about eating "Real Food".

What do you eat?

On my current nutrition plan I'm trying to put on size & lean mass without putting on too much excess fat. My meals consist of lean protein (egg whites, chicken breast, fish, turkey, and lean ground beef), low glycemic carbs (plain oatmeal, sweet potatoes, quinoa, brown rice), and good fats (MCT oil, olive oil, avocados, almond butter, mixed nuts raw no peanuts), and green vegetables.

My favorite recipe:

Pie Like Butternut Squash
Preheat oven to 400 degrees.
Take a butternut squash (oblong orange squash).
Cut it in ½ and remove the seeds.
Place face down in a glass cooking dish, with just a hint of water at the bottom. Cook approximately 45 minutes, or until soft. You can poke the outside with a fork to tell if it has softened. Once soft remove the squash, I then suggest letting it cool slightly. Remove the insides and place in a food processor (blender will work if you do not have one) add cinnamon and a pinch of nutmeg to taste. Puree until smooth. Let cool in the refrigerator, letting it sit overnight brings out more flavor. Take out and enjoy!

Do you take supplements?

I do take some supplements:
Kre-Alkalyn Creatine-to help my body recover from my workouts and help increase muscle mass.
Glutamine-protect muscle, help gut function, immune system, and body functions.
Omega Plex-General Wellness

What is your workout schedule and why?

My current workout schedule is lifting heavy & conditioning 6 days a week, abs 2x a week, and fasting cardio 3x a week.
My current goal is to increase lean muscle mass without putting on too much excess fat. So the heavy lifting with. help tear and rebuild my muscles to grow bigger and the cardio/conditioning will help trim. the excess fat. Food plays a major role in this too.

What is your definition of passion? Heart? Success?

My definition of passion is a strong feeling that you feel non stop and what drives you to do what you do everyday.

Heart just like your body is the center piece of everything you are doing. It's where your passion, dedication, will, values, and moral come from.

Everyone's definition of success is going to different. I believe success is consistency. Constant hard work, dedication, will, and never quitting just because there's struggles or lost battles. Keep moving forward, getting a little better everyday. Leaving an impact on others, that to me is success.

How do you stay motivated to make this a lifestyle and not a goal?

It's not an overnight deal to turn this from a goal to a lifestyle. A lot of my motivation comes from family at home and the people I work with at Integrity. Both are very supportive, understanding, and there when I need something. They're all different so I learn and take something from each one of their personalities, characters, and knowledge. My motivation also comes from my own passion for my clients and myself. When I see the changes not only in me but the clients. To see them happy for their accomplishments motivates me to keep doing what I do to help more people.

What does Train To Live mean to you?

Train To Live means don't just exist in this life but to live it. Take care of the body your were given so you can get the most out of life.

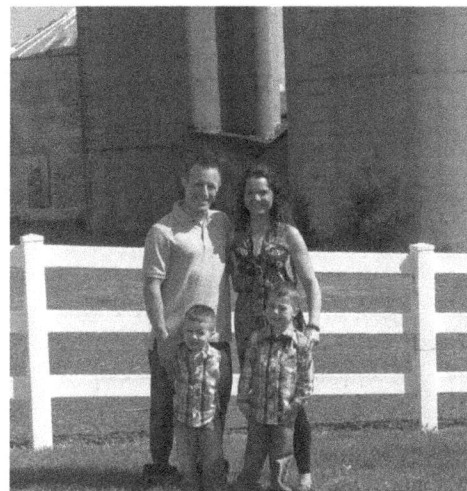
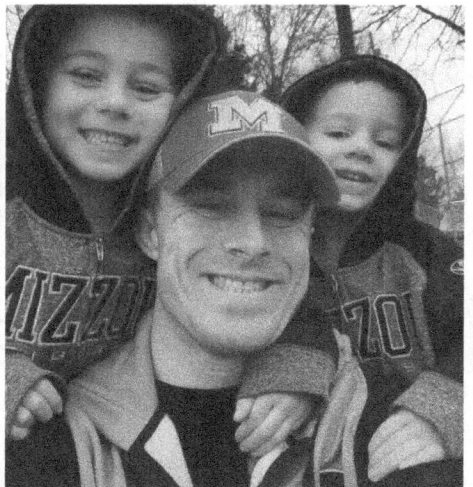
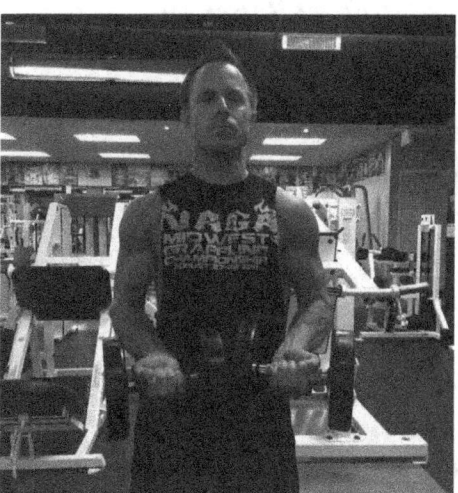

Workouts:
Legs:
2 Rounds of 10
Roman Deadlifts
Step Ups on Bench
Single Leg on Squat Sled
(10 each)
Sled Push/Pull 2x.

Next:
Leg Extension 15 every 15 seconds 4x
Leg Curls 15 every 15 seconds 4x

Next:
Squat Sled 30
Hack Squat 10
Swing Squat 10
Med ball squat pick up slam 10
Shoulders

4 Rounds:
Upright Cable Rows 10
V-Bar Front Raises 10
Rope Slams 20

Bosu Ball Arm Ups 10 each arm (modify on knees)

Next:
Iron Crosses 10
Thumb Out Bent Over Plys 10
Jump Rope 100
(modify invisible jump rope)
Chicken Wings 20
Chest

4 Rounds:
Cable Fly 10, Push ups 15

4 Rounds:
Incline Press 10, **Push ups** 15

4 Rounds: **Cable Fly Underneath** 10, **Push ups** 15

4 Rounds:
Cable Fly Top 10, **Push ups** 15
(No rest between set of 10 to push ups)

Arms
4 Rounds:
Overhead Rope Extensions 10
Cable Curl Bar 20
Weighted Dip -Machine 10
V Cable Curls 20
Then:
Hammer Curls 10
Cable Press Down 20
Cable Press Down 20
Reverse Curl 10
Reverse Tricep Extension 20

Back:
Wide Grip Cable Pull down 10
Close Grip Cable Row 20
Row Machine 1 min
Wide Grip Cable Row 10
Close Grip Cable Pull Down 20
Row Machine 1 min
Reverse Pee Dec 10
Bent Over Overhead Cable Pull-over 20
Row Machine 1 min

Cardio
8 Rounds of each exercise before moving to next one.

Work: *20 sec Rest: 10*
1 min rest between each new exercise

Work: *20 sec Rest: 10*
1 min rest between each new exercise

Flutter Kicks
Mt. Climbers
Ball Slams
Air Squats
Rope Slams
Reverse Crunch
Plank

Favorite Quotes:

"A river cuts through a rock not because of its power but its persistence." -Jim Watkins

"The two most important days in your life are the day you were born and the day you figure out why" -Mark Twain

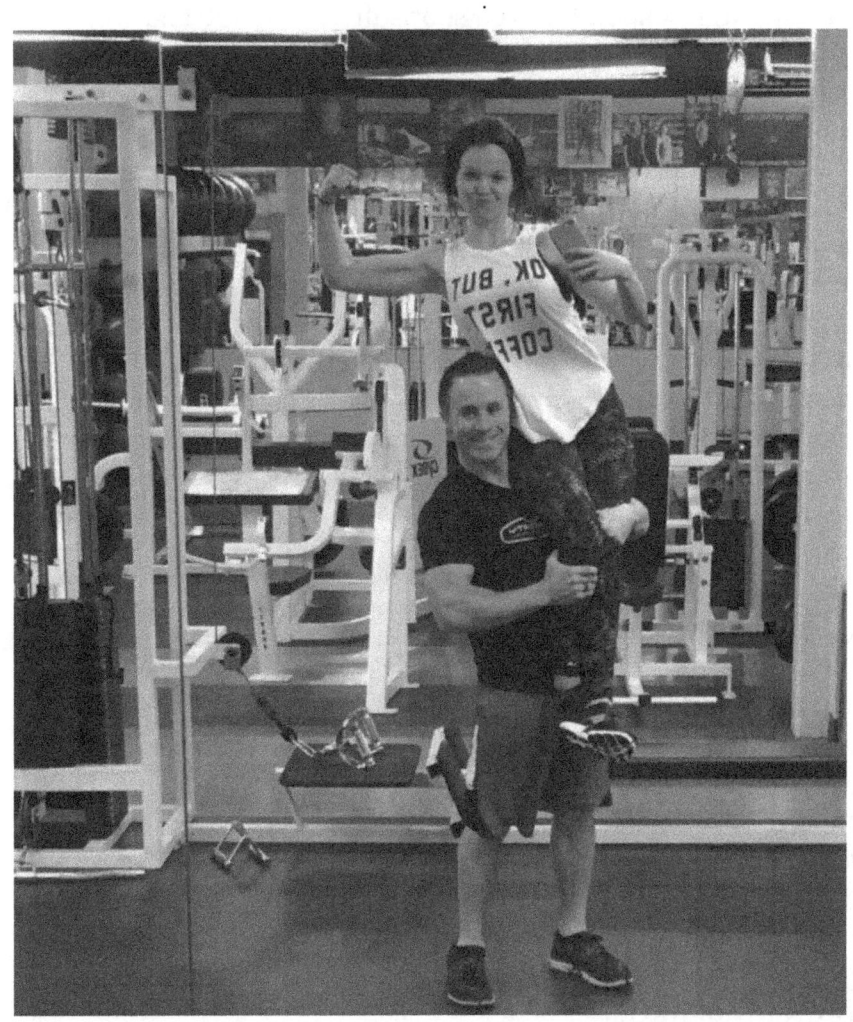

What made you a trainer?
Casey Owens

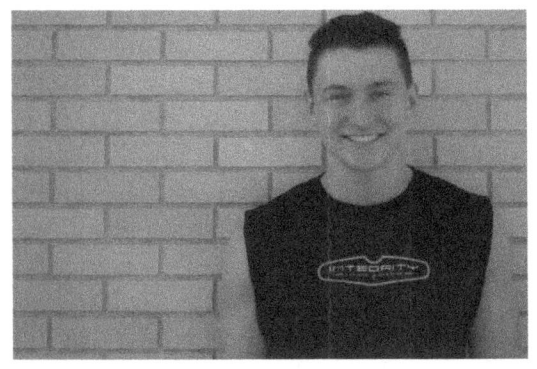

What really made me become a trainer was my mom. Ever since I was little I was always into sports and fitness related things always caught my attention and brought me the most joy. Whenever I was playing a sport or even working out in middle school and high school I always loved the way I felt and being able to push myself constantly. My passion for working out really took off about a year after high school. I played sports my whole life and when all of that ended I really felt like I was in a slump. One night while playing video games with a close buddy of mine he just stopped in the middle of everything and said "what are we doing". He also played sports his whole life and then I asked him what he meant. He wondered why we were just wasting our time away playing games instead of being active and getting in the gym. At this time it was also 1am. Right when he said that it really started to hit me that I needed to get back to the gym because I remembered what it felt like to be pushing myself and to be working towards some sort of goals. So from that moment on we told ourselves that we were getting back into the gym and we would hit it 6 days a week, every week. So at 1am we stopped playing video games and went straight to the gym. From that moment on I knew if I started that I would never want to finish. Fast forward about a year and a half and I was still going 6 days a week and trying to improve as much as I could. At this point my passion started to turn into trying to motivate others to pick up on this healthy lifestyle and get into the gym. What really help motivated me and made me so happy was seeing others transformations and reaching goals they never thought they could. My mom new this passion I had and so one day she came to me and

told me that she didn't think I was serious enough to get my nutrition on point and to start seeing Debbie for my nutrition. She told me I couldn't make it 2 weeks and anyone who knowns me knows that I don't back away from a challenge. My mom knows this and she knew I could do it but at the time she knew I needed that extra push because even though I hit the gym everyday my nutrition was horrible and it was really holding me back. So I started seeing Debbie and after 2 weeks I was in love with how amazing I felt and how much better I started to look. That's when I told Debbie that I wanted to compete in a men's physique bodybuilding show. I wanted to push my mind and body like I never have before and also stay dedicated to this lifestyle because my quality of life im-

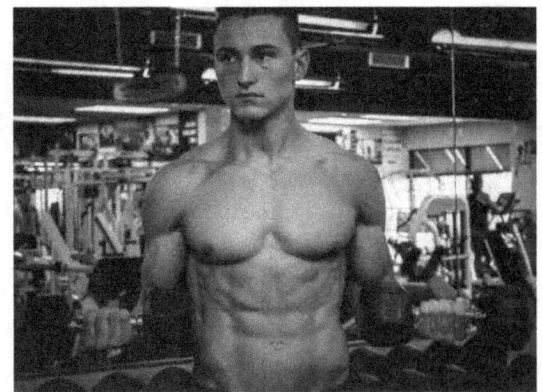

proved so drastically after I started feeding my body the proper foods. My mind was clearer, I went to bed and woke up easier, my acne started going away, I looked better and overall just felt way better. At the time I was going to school and I really wasn't sure which direction I wanted to go in life and every career I looked into just didn't set a spark in me. I knew about training and I would always think about how cool it would be to make my passion my profession and be able to help anyone I could. I didn't know much or where to start so I just always pushed it away. There was a job that I had an interview with and it was going to be a great job but I knew that each morning I was going to hate what I was doing and it would have felt like going through the same motions every day. About 2 months into dieting with Debbie and loving the healthy lifestyle Debbie stopped me one day and asked me what my plans in the future were. I told her I didn't know and there were several different jobs I was interested in but I really wasn't looking forward to any of them. So she asked me if I ever thought about being trainer. I told her yes but I never knew where to start or anything about it. Debbie in that moment started talking about it for 5 or 10 minutes and then offered me a job at Integrity. Right at that moment I knew that is what I wanted to do. If I could reach out to anyone I could and help them live a better life than I knew I would appreciate life and be in love with getting up every day and helping others. To me this isn't a job, I'm just doing what I love and that's all I have ever wanted. I was so excited and to this day I still wake up each morning excited with dedicating myself fully to this lifestyle. Even if I could help just one person's life then I would be truly happy. I am a trainer because I want to help others live a longer happier life and show them that through healthy eating and proper training that their quality of life will improve dramatically. I wake up each morning knowing that today I might touch someone's life and be able to help them get through with whatever problems they may be having at the time and that is what drives me and keeps me passionate every day. I would not want to choose life another way.

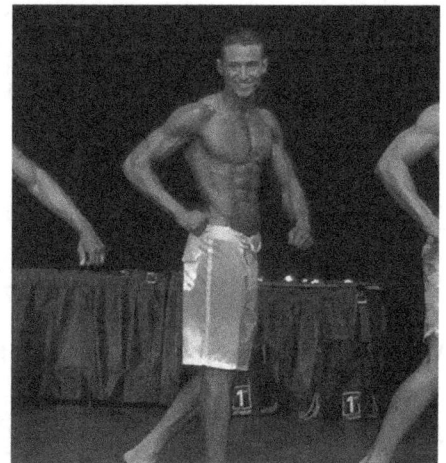

What are your strengths?

I'd have to say one of my strengths is being able to be open and talkative to new people. I love hearing what others have to say rather its negative or positive and just take whatever information I can from others and learn from it. You never know whose hand you are going to have the opportunity to shake one day so I'm grateful for all the new people I meet. Hearing stories and maybe having the ability to affect someone's life is what drives me.

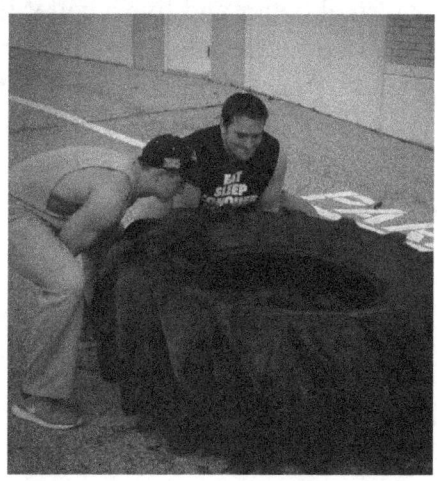

Weaknesses?

My biggest weakness I would have to say is always biting off more than I can normally chew. I tend to overload my mind and body just because I feel like I can always do more or be better than I was before. I love staying busy and having things to do but sometimes it can be a bit overwhelming. I look at it as I only have 24 hours so I should always try to fit as much stuff into my day as possible and keep myself busy.

What has your focus and what are your goals?

My main focus is always others, I want to help others with whatever possible and that is what I'm passionate about. I love seeing others make changes in their lives and living a happier life because of it. The more people I see change and grow for the better just keep motivating me and bring so much joy to me. I love seeing people live a happier life; it really does bring me true happiness. Never taking shortcuts and just taking one positive step at a time brings people true joy in life.

What is your philosophy on nutrition?

When it comes to nutrition I truly believe that you are what you eat so if you don't feel good or you are having different health issues then the first thing you need to look at is your DIET. Most of my days are personally filled with real chicken and organic sweet potatoes and I have no reason to complain about it. Most people ask me if I get sick of these foods and from time to time I may get tired of the taste but then I realize that I feel better and live a better life when I'm fueling myself with the correct foods. If I eat bad sugars or processed foods then I feel run down and sick to my stomach, why would I want to live life like that? Don't get me wrong I do treat myself but for a bulk of my diet I am eating healthy and getting the correct foods because I feel so much better doing so. I tend to be short on time with my schedule so the best way for me to cook my chicken is right from one of Debbie's recipes. I take one jar of bone sucking sauce and put 12 chicken breast into a crock pot and slow cook for 12 hours. Once that is done I drain the crock pot and then shred the chicken. I add one more bottle of bone sucking sauce and then I'm done. Most of my meal prepping is in bulk so that I have food all week long. Total time to prep all my food is maybe 1 hour at most. This is very easy and then I constantly have my meals all week long. You are what you eat so I always try to fuel my body with the proper nutrition.

My favorite recipe:

Debbie's Crockpot BBQ Chicken
One jar of bone sucking sauce
12 chicken breast
Put into a crock pot and slow cook for 12 hours. Once that is done I drain the crock pot and then shred the chicken. I add one more bottle of bone sucking sauce and then I'm done.

Most of my meal prepping is in bulk so that I have food all week long. Total time to prep all my food is maybe 1 hour at most. This is very easy and then I constantly have my meals all week long. You are what you eat so I always try to fuel my body with the proper nutrition.

Do you take supplements?

Supplements I take would consist glutamine, kre-alkayln, bcaas, and zmas. "Glutamine is produced in the muscles and is distributed by the blood to the organs that need it. Glutamine might help gut function, the immune system, and other essential processes in the body, especially in times of stress". " Kre-Alkalyn works by helping the body produce adenosine triphosphate, which is essential for energy transfer among cells. This increase of ATP production within the muscles creates increased energy for the athlete, which allows for longer, harder workouts". "It's well established that branched-chain amino acids (particularly leucine) stimulate protein synthesis, and might do so to a greater extent than a normal protein on its own. BCAAs also increase synthesis of the cellular machinery responsible for carrying out the process of protein synthesis". "ZMA is a natural mineral supplement made up of zinc, magnesium aspartate, and vitamin B6. Zinc supports your immune system and muscles. Magnesium plays a role in metabolism and muscle health and helps manage sleep. B6 may boost energy."

What is your workout schedule and why?

Currently my new workout schedule is a split routine with very heavy lifting. I am trying to grow a lot of muscle before I compete in another show next year. So I hit each muscle on different days and take only one rest day during the week. I do HIIT cardio 3 times a week before my first meal. I want to gain some muscle but I want to do it the right away and not gain a lot of fat. So I will eat a lot of clean food and hit cardio as well. This is going to be best for maximal muscle growth.

What is your definition of passion? Heart? Success?

Passion to me means having a desire for something so strong that most things will always come second to your passion. Passion is related to an addiction, it consumes your everyday life and that's all you think about and want all the time. You will do anything in your power to obtain it as well. Having heart to me means knowing what is right or wrong and you will be able to feel that within your heart. It will tell you what is wrong from right and always lead you into the positive direction. The heart and the human mind are so powerful together that I believe that people can accomplish anything they put their mind to if they truly believe they can do it. Listen to your heart and your gut and go after whatever it is you desire most in life. Being successful all comes down to your level of happiness in life. To me that is the only way it can be measured. If you are truly happy in life and love what you do then that is being successful. If you are not happy with your life or what you are doing then you need to go out and change that. Life is too short to be anything but happy so don't live an unhappy life. Do what makes you happy in life and I can promise you that everything will just seem to fall into place after that.

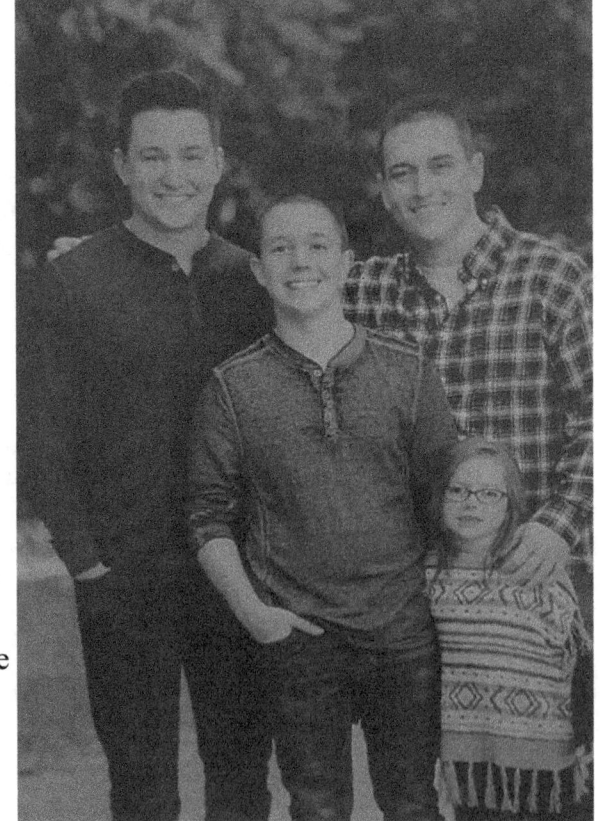

How do you stay motivated to make this a lifestyle and not a goal?

Keeping this lifestyle has become very easy. The moment I knew what I was doing right and what I was doing wrong was when I just started listening to my body. After eating clean all the time the moment I would eat something bad I could feel it affect my body for days after because my body hated the nasty processed food. I would feel tired, bloated, sick and just not myself. This was all because of eating a bad meal? Why would I want to feel that way? That's when I decided to make this my lifestyle. I won't lie because sometimes I will treat myself but on a daily basis I eat the right foods and train to stay healthy. I love the way I feel and that is what will make the quality of my life better every day. When I work out and eat healthy I feel great and have a positive mood and I also look better. I would much rather live my life feeling great and having a positive attitude instead of feeling down and depressed for something as little as "great tasting food". To me healthy food taste way better and processed foods are just way to strong and make you feel sick. I train and eat healthy to live the longest and the best life that I could possibly live.

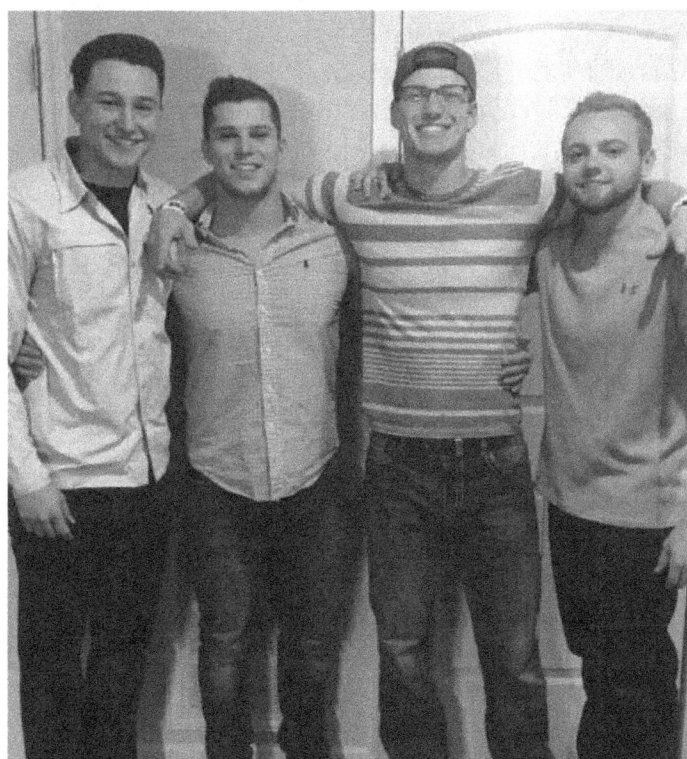
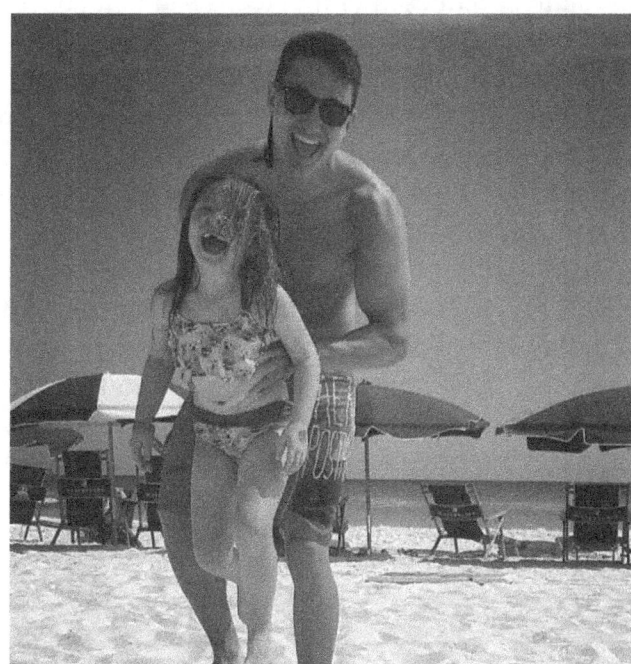

What does Train To Live mean to you?

Train to live, to me means to be always taking the right steps forward in your diet and training to enjoy life more often and to feel and look amazing while doing so.

Workouts that explain my style of training:

Right now my training consists of being body part specific. I am trying to gain the most muscle mass I can possible for when I compete next year in 2017. I do HIIT cardio 3x a week in the mornings before my first meal. I train triceps on Monday which consist of close grip bench, forward cable tri ext, overhead cable tri ext, barbell skull crusher and weighted dips. I do reps of 10,8,6,4,2. I finish my workout with hanging knees, bench crunch overhead floor crunch and torso twist crunch incline, dips, pull ups and pushups. All 100 reps each and then I do 1000 jump ropes. Tuesday I do my leg workout. This consist of squats, leg press, leg ext, lunge, Romanian dead lift, leg curl, seated calf raise all reps of 10,8,6,4,2. Then a slow burn for 10 min on the stairs. Wednesday I hit biceps and that consists of barbell curl, DB curl, DB hammer curl, cable double bicep, behind head cable curl and isolation DB curl. All reps of 10,8,6,4,2. Then I finish the workout with hanging knees, bench crunch, overhead floor crunch, torso twist crunch incline, dips, pullups and pushups. all 100 reps and then jump rope for 1000 reps. Thursday is my rest day. Friday I hit chest and that consist of decline press, bench press, and incline press, fly flat DB and cable fly mid. All reps of 10,8,6,4,2. Then I finish the lift with pullups, pushups each 100 reps and jump rope for 1000 reps. Saturday I train back and that consist of deadlift, tbar row, bent over row, seated cable row, wide lat pull down and bent over DB fly. All reps of 10,8,6,4,2. Then I finish the lift with pull ups and pushups, each 100 reps and then jump ropes for 1000 reps. Last is Sunday and I train shoulders. That day consist of DB knuckle out press, Arnold press, standing barbell military press, upright row from the ground, standing DB lateral raise, iron cross and chicken wings. Reps of 10,8,6,4,2. Then I finish with pull ups and pushups 100 reps each and jump ropes for 1000 reps. This has been my weekly routine at the time being but it does change! This is for trying to grow the most muscle mass I can. I also do foam rolling and stretching at least twice a day, once in the morning and before my lifts.

Favorite Quotes:

"A well built physique is a status symbol. It reflects you worked hard for it, no money can buy it. You cannot borrow it, you cannot inherit it, you cannot steal it. You cannot hold onto it without constant work. It shows discipline, it shows self respect, it shows patience, work ethic and passion. That is why I do what I do." -Arnold Schwarzenegger

"A dream doesn't become reality through magic; it takes sweat, determination and hard work." -Colin Powell

"Your mind is a powerful thing. When you fill it with positive thoughts, your life will start to change".

Why should you choose Integrity?

Why you should choose integrity is simple. When you join our group that makes you apart of the family. Its not only about losing weight or reaching your goals, its about becoming close and bringing you in as another family member. We care for all the things that you do in your life and even hitting the goals outside the gym. We all care for each other like a family does and that is what makes us unique. So to me its more about choosing us as a family and don't look at us as only a "gym" because everyone means more to us that just a client. That's why you should choose integrity, family always first.

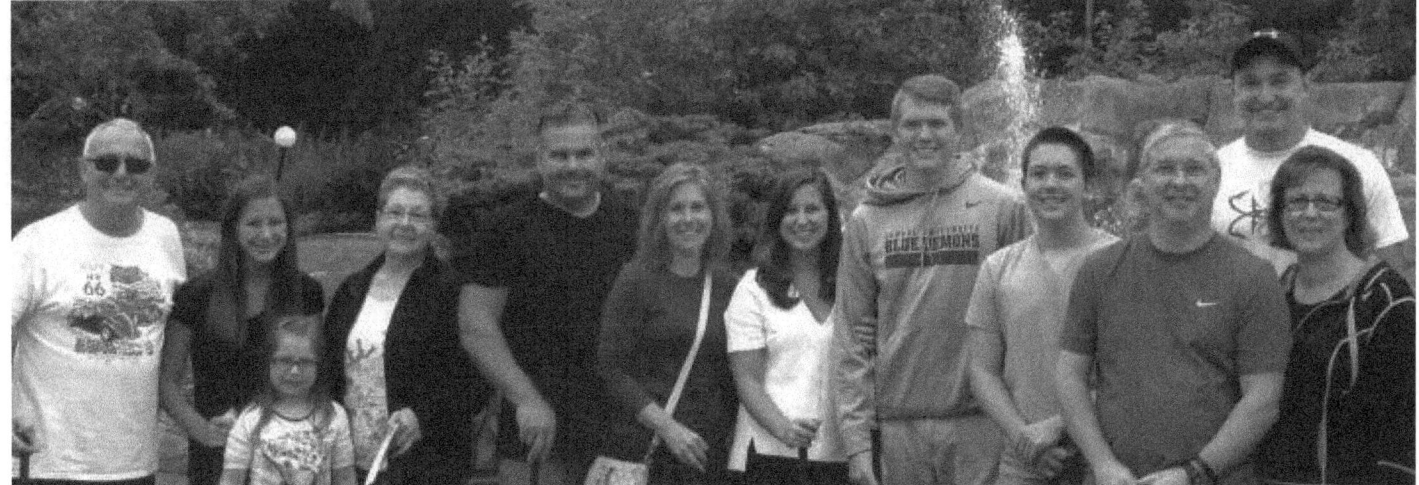

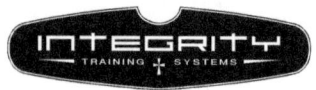

Debbie Portell
636.299.2208
[e]: debbiecooperportell@yahoo.com
www.integritytraininggroup.com
www.debbieportell.com

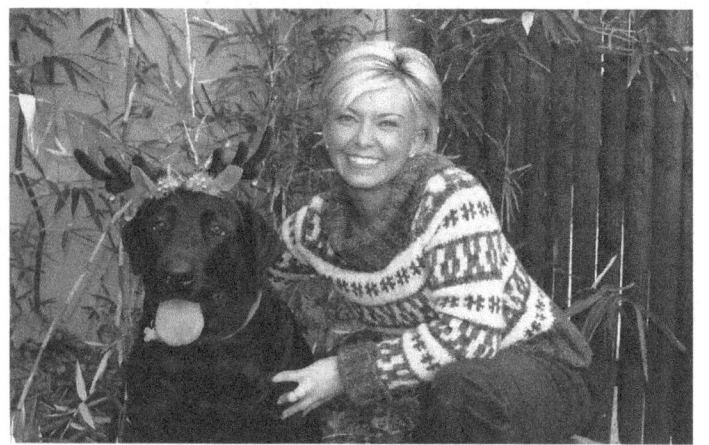
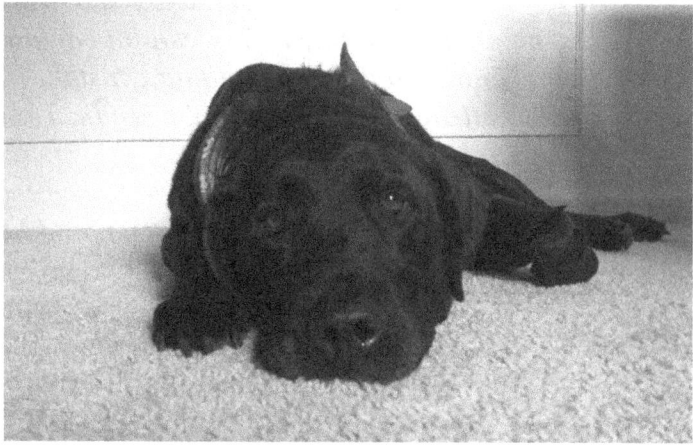

"I can do all things through Christ who strengthens me."
-Philippians 4:13

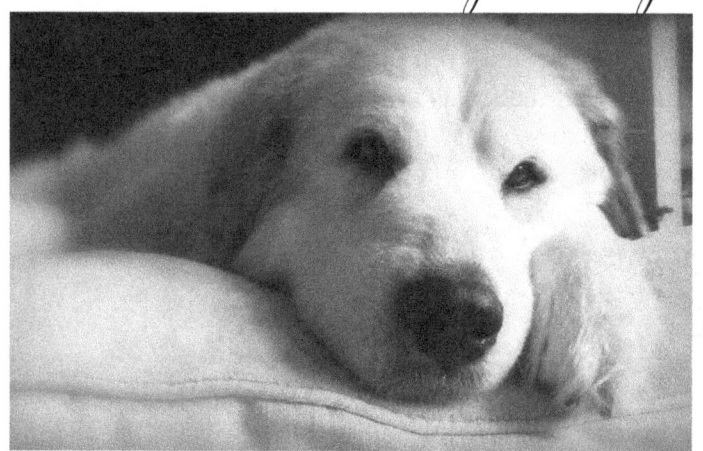
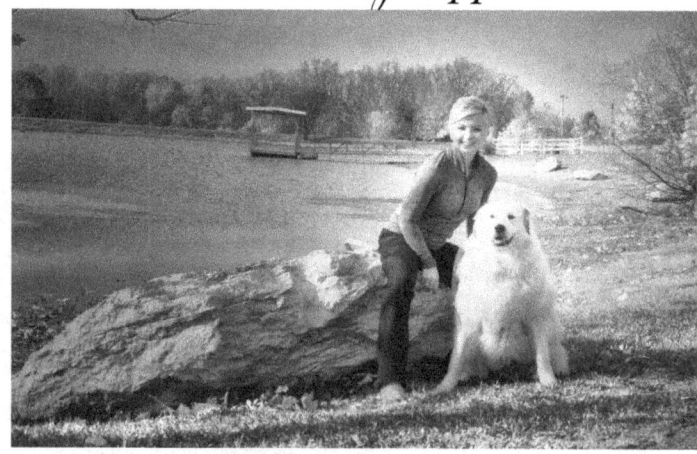

Without Him we can do nothing